# IITK Directions

## Volume 7

**IITK Directions** is an institutional series of the Indian Institute of Technology Kanpur. IITK Directions aims at presenting original contributions and reviews of important and cutting-edge topics by the faculty members and other stakeholders of IIT Kanpur in a consolidated manner. It is a platform that reflects upon the ongoing research and development activities, major achievements, and evolving trends. Each volume in the series focuses on a particular area of science and technology with chapters written by the faculty members, students and research staff. Each chapter is written in a journalistic tone for the peer group – readability and accessibility being important parameters. The volumes contain a survey of the subject as a whole and the extent of contributions recorded by the Institute faculty and students who participate so extensively in research.

The volumes in this series will be useful to researchers, practitioners, students, industry leaders, government officials and policy makers. Above all, the series serves as platform to publish the most cutting edge research summaries and evaluate the applications and impact of the research work undertaken at IIT Kanpur.

Sandeep Verma
Editor

# Technology and Innovation in Medical Sciences

## Breakthroughs from Gangwal School of Medical Sciences and Technology, IIT Kanpur

Springer

*Editor*
Sandeep Verma
Gangwal School of Medical Sciences
and Technology
Indian Institute of Technology Kanpur
Kanpur, Uttar Pradesh, India

ISSN 2509-6591 ISSN 2509-6605 (electronic)
IITK Directions
ISBN 978-981-96-8605-6 ISBN 978-981-96-8606-3 (eBook)
https://doi.org/10.1007/978-981-96-8606-3



This Springer imprint is published by the registered company Springer Nature Singapore Pte Ltd.
The registered company address is: 152 Beach Road, #21-01/04 Gateway East, Singapore 189721, Singapore

## Series Editor's Preface

I feel elated about this special issue of Directions, which delves into a broad spectrum of groundbreaking technology and innovations in Medical Science and Technology being developed at the upcoming Gangwal School of Medical Sciences and Technology. At this juncture, I would also like to shed light on the genesis of this issue.

IIT Kanpur has a rich legacy of successfully implementing innovative strategies in education, technology, and research projects that have a significant impact on society. One particularly ambitious initiative from IIT Kanpur is the Gangwal School of Medical Sciences and Technology, where technological advancements are set to propel future innovations in medicine and healthcare. With its rich history, capabilities and facilities in MedTech Innovation, IIT Kanpur aims to close the existing gap by founding a unique Medical School that will facilitate a transformative approach to medical research and MedTech innovation in the country.

This volume will explore the dynamic intersection of medicine and technology, emphasizing innovative advancements and their impact on healthcare. It addresses a wide array of subjects, such as the concept of digital twins, assistive and point-of-care health devices, the development and utilization of engineered materials, and the development of indigenous left ventricular assist devices (LVAD) and percutaneous ventricular assist devices (PVAD), emphasizing local efforts to advance cardiac care. Additionally, it explores optical tools in healthcare, covering recent progress in imaging, diagnostics, and minimally invasive surgical methods.

I extend my thanks to the authors for their willing contributions of the articles. I also express my appreciation to the editor and the publication team for enhancing the overall quality of the publication. Drawing on my previous experiences with earlier issues of Directions, I anticipate achieving an even broader reach with this specific issue, and I am confident that readers will acknowledge the value of the two-stage editing process.


Prof. Tarun Gupta<br>
Dean, Research and Development<br>
IIT Kanpur<br>
Kanpur, India

# Contents

## About the Editor

**Prof. Sandeep Verma** is currently heading the Gangwal School of Medical Sciences and Technology (GSMST) at the Indian Institute of Technology (IIT) Kanpur. His academic training has been achieved at University of Illinois (Ph.D.) and postdoctoral training at Johns Hopkins Medical Institutions and Max-Planck-Institute for Experimental Medicine. With over two hundred forty publications, several book chapters, multiple patents, and a biotechnology start-up to his credit, his work has been recognized by top scientific awards that include Shanti Swarup Bhatnagar Prize, Gold Medal (SMC-BARC), Swarnajayanti Fellowship, and Distinguished Alumnus Award of Banaras Hindu University, to name a few. Prof. Verma is also an elected Fellow of all four academies of science and engineering of India: INSA, INAE, IASc, and NASI. At the international level, Prof. Verma holds Honorary Professorships at two Australian universities and is currently providing leadership as a Member, Executive Board, Commonwealth Chemistry, Federation of Commonwealth Chemical Societies, UK.

One of his most significant and relevant past roles was as Secretary of the Science and Engineering Research Board (SERB) at the Department of Science and Technology, India, from 2019–2022. It involved planning, promotion, funding, and support of internationally competitive research in emerging areas of science and engineering. Prof. Verma was a Member of Prime Minister Office' Taskforce for SARS Cov-2 Vaccine, DST sub-committee on SARS diagnostics, and Empowered Group-1 on Emergency Management Plan and Strategy for COVID-19. He has also been actively engaged as a Governing Board member of IISER Bhopal and Berhampur, Indo-US Science and Technology Forum and Indo-German Science and Technology Center, New Delhi.

# Technology-Driven Academic and R&D Innovations in Medical Sciences

**1**

Deepashree Sheshadri and Sandeep Verma

**Abstract**

Indian Institute of Technology Kanpur (IIT Kanpur) has established a new medical school to bring a paradigm shift toward medical research and innovation in the country and bridge the gap between medical sciences and technology. With 75 years of proven excellence in engineering and technological education at IIT Kanpur and having one of the best innovation and incubation ecosystems, setting up of Gangwal School of Medical Sciences and Technology (GSMST) ushers a futuristic vision of an engineering-infused academic curriculum for post-graduate super-speciality medical disciplines and technology-driven biomedical science and MedTech innovations. GSMST will bring together available expertise of IIT Kanpur's faculty across science, engineering and humanities disciplines to address the unmet challenges. These endeavors are supported through intramurally funded R&D Centers of Excellence (CoE). These R&D CoE are specialized centers in targeted biomedical research areas and proposed to work with core clinical departments of super-speciality hospital, including cardiology, neurology, gastroenterology and nephrology, to train and nurture next-generation medical practitioners and medical engineers to develop solutions for equitable healthcare.

**Keywords**

MedTech · Healthcare innovation · Biomedical R&D · Clinical medicine · Post-graduate medical program

## 1.1 Premise

Advances in medical technology are poised to promote the transformation of healthcare delivery toward improved health outcomes. Digital healthcare ecosystem trends such as telemedicine, artificial intelligence, IoT-based wearable devices, augmented and virtual reality, medical drones, digitization of medical records, and blockchain in healthcare, will reshape and reimagine healthcare. The impact of technology-driven healthcare will demand innovation in diagnosis and treatment. Advanced treatment regimes such as telehealth, remote patient monitoring, robotic surgery, gene therapy, precision medicine, evidence-based medicine, and non-invasive diagnosis supported by AI, etc., will revolutionize healthcare. Thus, it is clear that strengthening digital healthcare through technology-infused medical delivery will disrupt the healthcare landscape.

In the Indian context, disruptions ushered through engineering-driven medicine could also be aligned with the mandates prescribed by the National Medical Commission (NMC) of India are (i) improve access to quality and affordable medical education, (ii) ensure availability of adequate and high-quality medical professionals; (iii) promote equitable and universal healthcare; (iv) encourage medical professionals to adopt latest medical research and to contribute to research [1]. Similarly, the mandate of the National Board of Examinations (NBE) is to empower and enrich human resources in medical sciences by providing robust, innovative, low-cost post-graduate teaching programs to ensure the highest standards of healthcare and

D. Sheshadri · S. Verma (✉)
Gangwal School of Medical Sciences and Technology, Indian Institute of Technology Kanpur, Kanpur, India
e-mail: sverma@iitk.ac.in


S. Verma (ed.), *Technology and Innovation in Medical Sciences*, IITK Directions 7,
https://doi.org/10.1007/978-981-96-8606-3_1

make India a hub of highly skilled and knowledgeable specialist doctors who can work across the urban–rural divide to provide best specialist care [2].

### 1.1.1 Global Healthcare Transformation

The future of global healthcare sector is poised for profound changes. It is likely to be shaped by open innovation, sustainable practices, integration of cost-effective social care, cost management, and technology adaptation [3]. Advancements in medical engineering and technology will be a key driver to shape the future of healthcare and medical education in India and globally. The COVID-19 pandemic set into motion a digital revolution in pedagogy, which will extend to simulation-based digital interventions for medical teaching and learning.

India has ~4.6 million healthcare resources (doctors, nurses and midwives), with a density of 33.5 per 10,000 population, which is significantly lower than many developed nations such as USA (183), UK (118.6), Brazil (97.1) and China (53.1) [4]. India has a shortfall of ~40,000 doctors, with 9 doctors per 10,000 population, compared with the WHO recommended density of 10 per 10,000 [4]. Thus, there is an immediate need to bridge the gap, and use innovative healthcare models and technology is the need of the hour.

The intersection of healthcare and technology will play an important and innovative role in shaping the future of healthcare. In addition, research breakthroughs in biomedical and bioengineering with emerging technologies, including in-silico protein folding prediction, novel cell therapies and other technology-driven treatment platforms, will further support quality healthcare delivery. Medical technology will also be a unique disruptor for rural and remote healthcare delivery.

### 1.1.2 Disruption in Healthcare Through Digital Technology

The government of India has transformed digital healthcare using Aarogya Setu, National Health Stack (NHS), National eHealth Authority (NeHA) and e-Sanjeevani [5]. Digital health-driven transformation is needed to reconfigure India's current healthcare system. With the advent of advanced technologies, enormous healthcare data and the advent of medical devices, including sensors, wearables, and implantables, clinicians are poised to track patient's health better. Further, advances in artificial intelligence (AI) and medical robotics are paving the way toward technology informed medical regime leveraged for diagnosis and treatment. Increased penetration of telehealth also pushes access and delivery of healthcare services to patients' doorstep, especially for remote locations [6].

Some of these advanced technologies support modern treatment and diagnostic options such as minimally invasive and high-precision robotic surgeries, Big Data in healthcare, advanced gene therapy, and precision personalized medicine. These interventions will rely on a paradigm shift toward "Digital Pathology," which entails high-resolution and magnification scanning of all pathology observations, followed by accurate, precise, and thorough annotation of scanned images using data sources and levels of clinical and pathological (gross pathology, histopathology, and molecular) information.

### 1.1.3 Technology-Infused Medical Program

Although the transdisciplinary R&D ecosystem fosters the growth of biomedical research and MedTech developments, most medical institutions in India and worldwide still follow a "stand-alone" approach. The latter is compounded by lack of involvement of professionals from non-medical fields, specialists focused on research, and a high patient load preventing doctors from actively participating in innovative translational research. Thus, a significant knowledge gap exists in medical education, MedTech innovation and entrepreneurship activity.

It is emphasized that technological interventions will drive future advancements in medicine and healthcare. This necessitates integration of technology and research knowledge into the medical education system. World-class universities such as Harvard-MIT Program in Health Sciences and Technology (HST), Duke-NUS Medical School, Stanford research ecosystem, and the University of Illinois Carle College of Medicine (UIUC) are exemplary models for Futuristic Medical Programs, which is currently not available in India.

## 1.2 Genesis of Biomedical Teaching and Research at IIT Kanpur

Engineering solutions play an integral role in biomedical sciences. The Indian Institute of Technology Kanpur (IIT Kanpur) has a large pool of academic expertise and considering the importance of the interface of biology and engineering in future medicine, several departments and centers such as Biological Sciences and Bioengineering, Physics, Material Science Engineering (MSE), Mechanical Engineering (ME), Chemistry, Computer Science Engineering, Electrical Engineering, BIRAC Center for Fabrication and Testing of Medical Devices, Center for Experimental Animal Facility, Centre for Cybersecurity, Center for Lasers and Photonics, Center for Nanoscience, DBT School for Healthcare Innovation and Entrepreneurship, ICMR CoE in Medical Research, National Center for Flexible Electronics (NCFlexE), Start-up Incubation and Innovation Centre (SIIC), Mehta Family Center for Engineering Medicine (MFCEM), are playing strong emphasis on biomedical research.

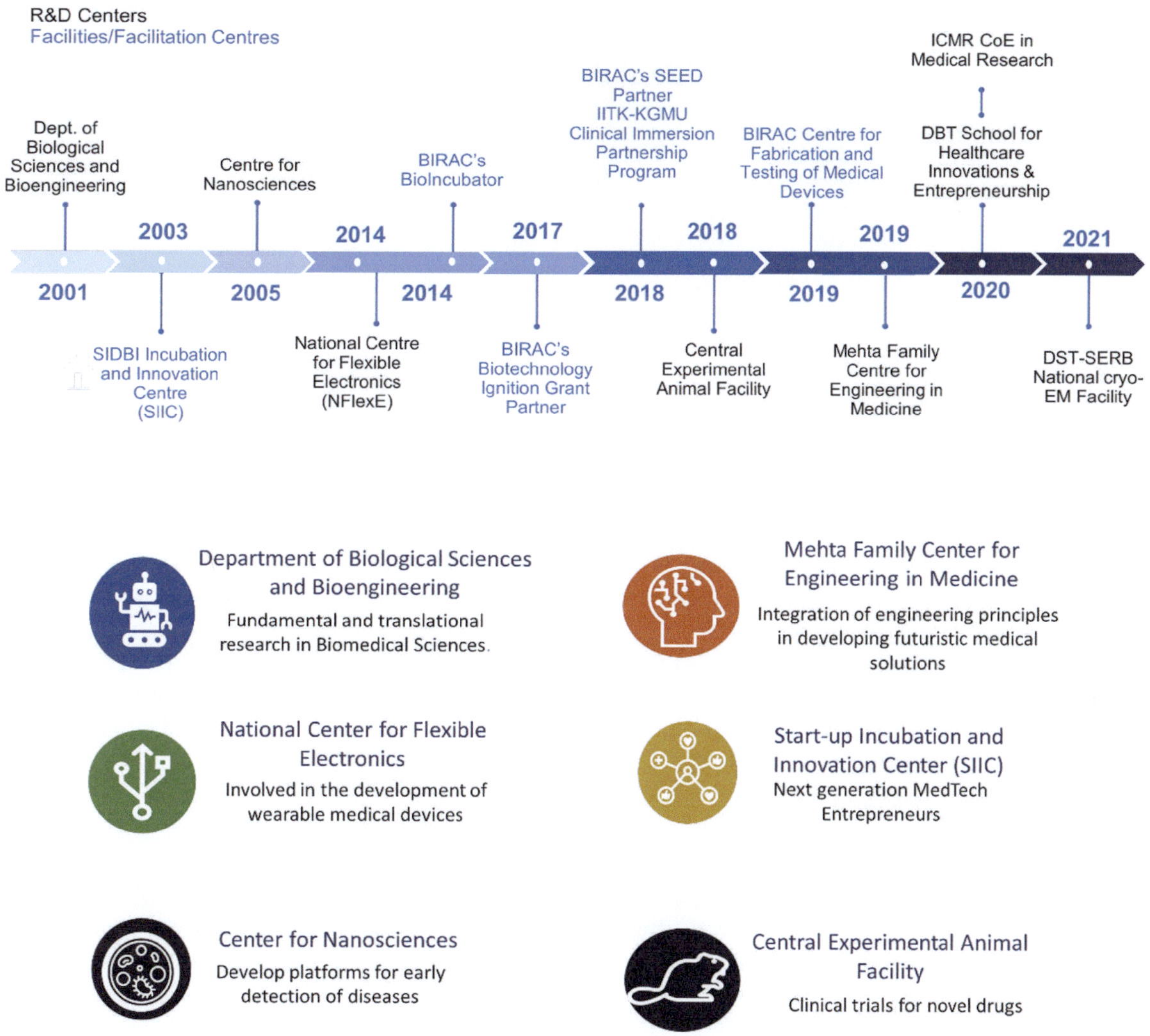


IIT Kanpur established the Department of Biological Sciences and Bioengineering (BSBE) in 2001, which offers B.Tech, M.Tech and PhD programs in many sub-disciplines. The Institute has established a strong innovation and incubation ecosystem, with a world-class incubation center with multiple success stories and one of the highest patent-to-commercialization ratio. The Institute has established a fabrication and certification center for MedTech devices and a state-of-the-art experimental animal facility for pre-clinical studies, thus attracting funding from the Department of Biotechnology to set up a School of Biodesign to promote innovation and entrepreneurship activities in the biomedical domain.

With the launch of several new initiatives, IIT Kanpur has earned a formidable name in medical research and MedTech innovations. DST, DBT and ICMR, have invested in R&D through the creation of required infrastructure for pre-clinical research, prototype and testing facility, and manpower development in allied areas. However, the lack of an on-campus academic program in medicine and clinical set-up hampers the progress in MedTech innovation and clinical research space in the Institute.

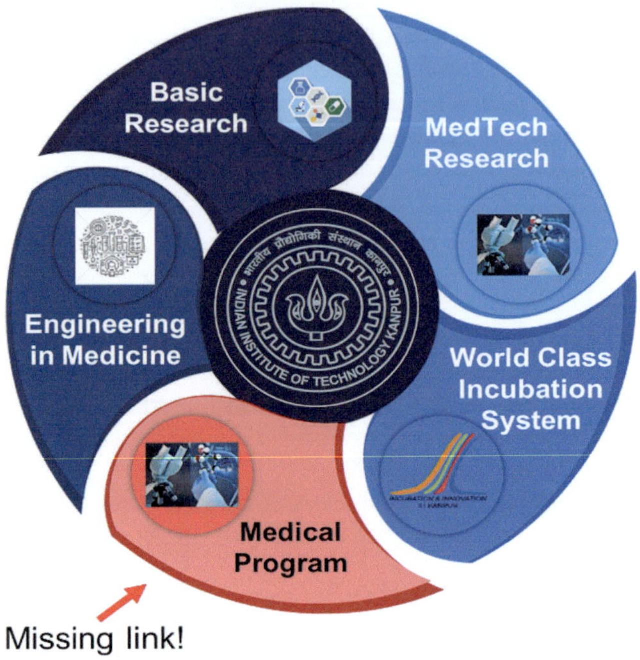


To evolve a transdisciplinary ecosystem for MedTech innovation and to bridge the gap between medicine and engineering in product-orientated collaborative research, the Institute presented a concept note for establishing a Medical School that specializes in high-end medical/clinical research involving contemporary science and engineering approaches for MedTech innovation and to offer academic programs in medicine and allied areas. Consequently, Gangwal School of Medical Sciences and Technology (GSMST) was established at IIT Kanpur," which will enable engineering and technology driven medical education and clinical research. Such an approach also aligns well with National Education Policy (NEP) 2020 which mandates transformation of Higher Education Institutions into large, well-resourced, vibrant multidisciplinary institutions. National Health Policy 2017 also aims to achieve universal access to quality healthcare through better-trained human resources, new knowledge and disruptive technologies.

## 1.3 Vision of GSMST

IIT Kanpur established GSMST with the objective of bringing a paradigm shift in the content and delivery of medical education, biomedical and clinical research, and MedTech innovation by bridging the gap between medical sciences, engineering and technology.

- train next-generation medical practitioners and medical engineers.
- develop affordable devices and technologies for medical/healthcare needs.
- develop engineering solutions for unmet medical needs.
- serve as hub for healthcare technology.
- serve as a model for technology-driven medical institutions.

### 1.3.1 Structure and Components of GSMST

GSMST design involves IIT Kanpur's faculty, cutting across traditional disciplines built around a super-speciality hospital, biomedical research prowess, and various R&D Centers of Excellence (CoE). These CoEs will specialize in niche biomedical research areas and are expected to work in tandem with core clinical departments of the Medical School and hospital and bring in biomedical expertise from various engineering, science and humanities departments of IIT Kanpur.

The School will have three main components:

1. **Academics**: School plans to focus on super-speciality post-graduate medical programs like DM and MCh (regular medical stream) and transdisciplinary research programs (MD/MS-PhD) in engineering/science/medicine interface areas. Apart from super-speciality post-graduate programs, nursing and paramedical School are also envisaged. A non-medical joint degree program on "Healthcare Management" has also been initiated with IIM Lucknow.
2. **Hospital Complex**: This complex includes a 500-bed super-speciality hospital and a 100-bedded Cancer Care and Research Center, with a world-class facility on board, which will offer affordable treatment in specialities like oncology, cardiology, cardiothoracic surgery, nephrology, neurology, neurosurgery, etc. to over 4 million people in and around Kanpur and connected region.
3. **R&D Centers of Excellence (CoE)**: CoE bring together the strength of IIT Kanpur faculty, cutting across disciplines such as science, engineering, and humanities, to leverage biomedical research and MedTech innovation. The eventual goal is to make the School one of the top destinations for MedTech Innovation and to provide technological solutions for unmet healthcare needs.

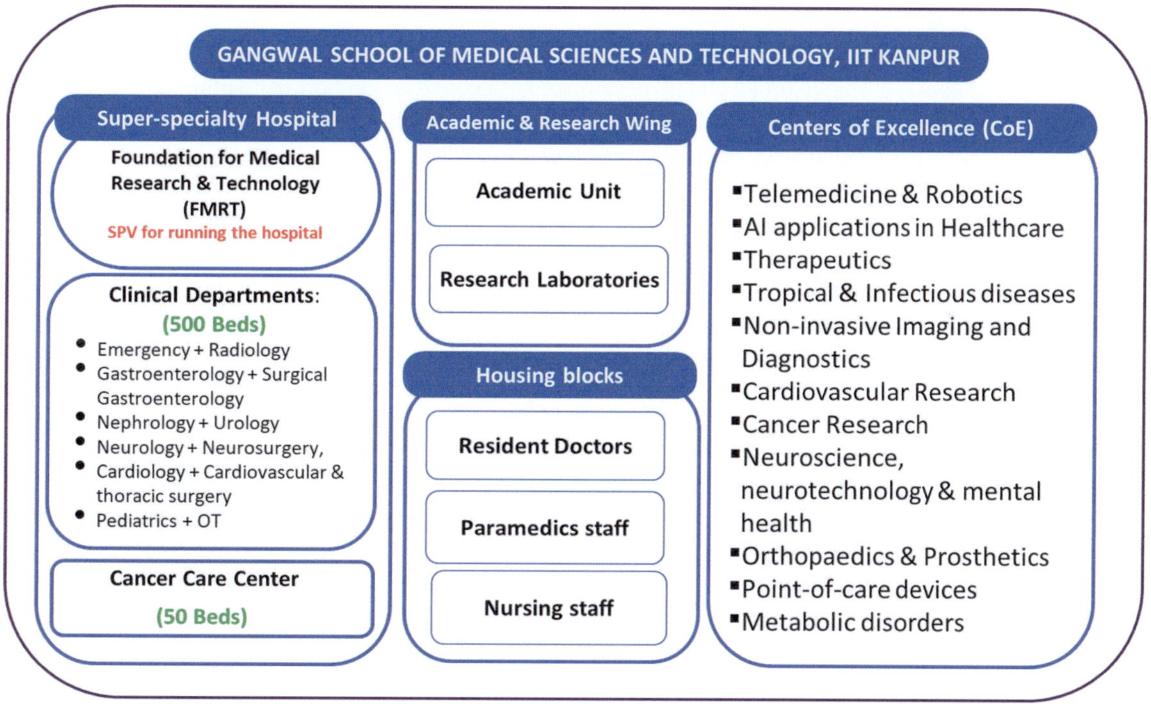


### 1.3.2 Infrastructure Planning

Phase I of the School will be built over a 30-acre plot within the IIT Kanpur campus, with spaces planned for academic, research and clinical components. First phase of the project focuses on establishing a super-speciality hospital, an oncology block, and necessary supporting infrastructure, including engineering and ancillary services block.

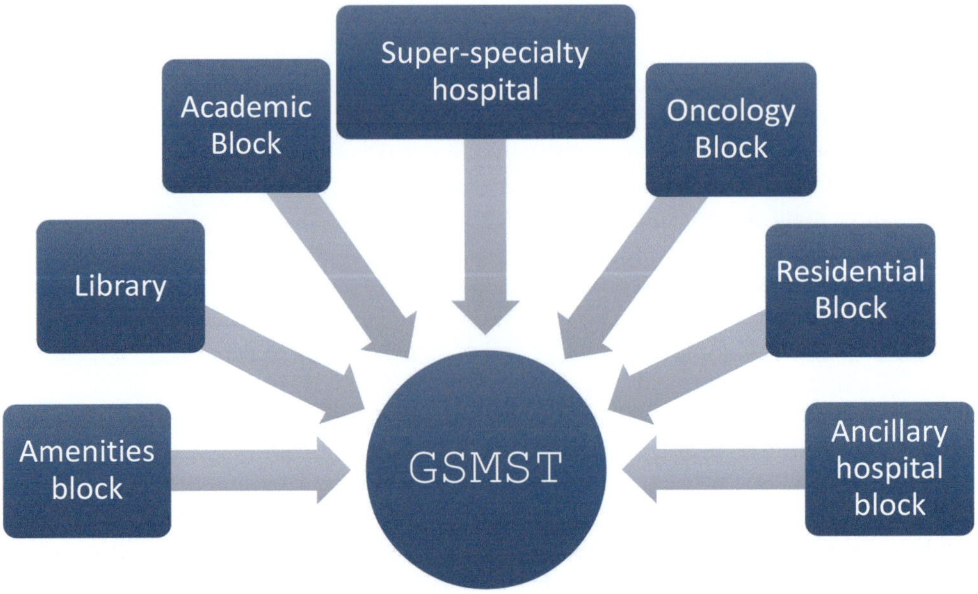


### 1.3.3 Fundraising Activities

IIT Kanpur Medical School is a unique project being developed with generous support from philanthropists, IITK alumni and corporates. The Institute is seeking funding from alumni, corporates, and philanthropists to develop the project. The Institute has already initiated a process to attract funding for research and innovation.

Shri Rakesh Gangwal, a Distinguished Alumnus of the Institute, generously donated toward the infrastructure and building of the School. For his contribution, the School is named **"Gangwal School of Medical Sciences and Technology."** Further, Mr Muktesh Pant, Dr Dev Joneja, Shri Hemant Jalan, and Shri Anil Bansal have committed to donating to establish the School as part of the Founder's Circles of GSMST. Institute has also received the commitment for the super-speciality hospital (JK Cement Ltd), administrative and academic blocks, and the residential block. Recently, the Government of Uttar Pradesh committed to supporting the construction of the super-speciality hospital.

### 1.3.4 Foundation Stone Laying Ceremony

The Union Minister of Education and Skill Development and Entrepreneurship, Shri Dharmendra Pradhan, laid the foundation stone of the Gangwal School of Medical Sciences and Technology and the Yadupati Singhania Super-Speciality Hospital at the IIT Kanpur campus on 16th July 2022 by unveiling the plaques. The ceremony was presided over by Dr K Radhakrishnan, Chairman, Board of Governors, IIT Kanpur.

### 1.3.5 Research and Development with Centers of Excellence in GSMST

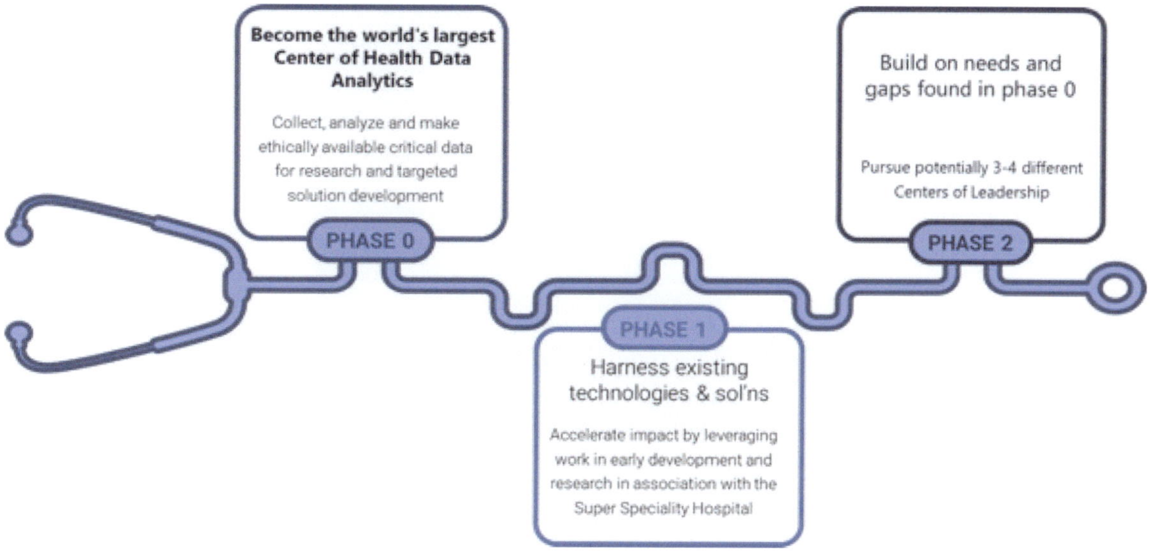


The Hospital will be the confluence of IIT Kanpur's faculty, cutting across the disciplines built on the backbone of a super-speciality hospital and various centers of excellence. These CoE will be specialized centers in targeted biomedical research areas and are expected to work in confluence with core clinical departments of medical School and biomedical expertise of various engineering departments of IIT Kanpur. A concise blueprint of phase-wise R&D activities has been defined. CoE themes are both unique and multidisciplinary in nature. For example, *CoE in Artificial Intelligence in Healthcare* seeks to develop state-of-the-art machine learning algorithms capable of providing clinical decision support to doctors, enabling them to reach a larger population of patients on a day-to-day basis; *CoE in Cardiovascular and Pulmonary Disease Research* aims to come with low-cost medical support devices like LVAD, IV-LITHOTRIPSY, heart valves, pacemakers; *CoE in Non-invasive Imaging and Diagnostics* focuses on developing improved imaging technologies, novel measurement configurations, data interpretation algorithms for improved diagnostics, and specialized instrumentation; *CoE in Telemedicine and Robotics* aims to develop an array of surgical, diagnostic, telepresence, exoskeleton robots and simulating platforms; *CoE in Therapeutics* aims to discover, develop and deliver novel, affordable and scalable therapies for tropical diseases, inherited diseases, cancer, infectious diseases and immunological disorders; *CoE in Neuroscience, neurotechnology and mental health* will focus on systems for automated analysis of neural data, diagnostic systems for brain disorders, tools for neurosurgery, and development of brain-computer interfaces; *CoE in Materials in Medicine* will cater to comprehensive and multidisciplinary advancements required for musculoskeletal diseases and trauma; *CoE in Tropical and Infectious Diseases* will target technological advancement and development of diagnostics, therapeutics and preventive methods; and *CoE in Cancer Research* focuses on nuclear medicines, cancer immunotherapy, point-of-care devices and sensors, genomic or transcriptomic studies, to name a few.

- AI in Healthcare
- Cancer Research
- Cardiovascular & Pulmonary disease research
- Metabolic Disorders
- Neuroscience, Neurotechnology & Mental Health
- Non-invasive medical imaging & Diagnostics
- Materials in medicine
- Point-of-care diagnostics
- Therapeutics
- Telemedicine & Robotics
- Tropical & infectious diseases

CoE in Cardiovascular and Pulmonary Diseases Research has launched an ambitious multidisciplinary project, ‘Hridyantra’, developing a new generation Indigenous **Left Ventricular Assist device (LVAD)**. This indigenous device is well progressing toward animal trials. IIT Kanpur team, along with expert clinicians, aim to develop superior-performing, better hemocompatible, and low-cost LVAD, making its implantation affordable to a substantially greater fraction of people suffering from end-stage heart failure.

Four "Flagship Projects" and two "Proof-of-concept" technology demonstrators are currently under advanced stages of investigation:

**Flagship projects**

- Self-navigating smart wheelchair
- Percutaneous mechanical circulatory support systems
- Single optical fiber-based endoscope
- 3D printed interbody spacer with nanoparticles for spinal deformity

**Proof-of-concept technology demonstrators**

- Rapidly deployable cardiac digital twin
- Technology platform for eradication of bacteria by plasmonic heating

### 1.3.6 Impact of the Gangwal School of Medical Sciences and Technology

The Gangwal School, housing a 500+ bedded super-speciality/ tertiary care hospital with state-of-the-art medical technology, will have 50% beds designed and modeled to cater to government-financed health coverage scheme patients.

*Digital Health Stack and Medical Device Reforms*—GSMST will provide insights to digital health sector to to align with the requirements of National Digital Health Mission (NDHM). A pilot project involving Uttar Pradesh government has already been initiated and our efforts will continue to drive innovation in the digitization of Indian healthcare data and integration to national mission, telemedicine, remote health management, personal health monitoring devices, and other digital technology-driven care system models.

A partnership with Uttar Pradesh Government has led to the creation of hybrid Digital Health Stack for UP (DHS-UP), augmenting physical PHC and CHC networks in the state with a suite of digital technologies to enable both private and public health service providers. Researchers from IIT Kanpur are working closely with health department of the state to create digital health stack for disease projections, surveillance, and supply chains.

*UP Clinical Trials Group*—As part of UP Government (Medical Education Department-2) Clinical Trials Group, Gangwal School of Medical Sciences and Technology will strengthen the importance of clinical trials in affordable product development and market transfer.

*Access to new and emerging medical technology*—The interdisciplinary clinical research programs at the Gangwal School will address a variety of ailments, including diabetes, metabolic disorders, neurodegenerative diseases, cancer, cardiovascular diseases, and infectious diseases such as Tuberculosis, HIV, and COVID-19.

- The focus would be to understand underlying molecular mechanisms of diseases and develop affordable solutions for diagnostics and therapies.
- Advancements in communication technologies (5G and beyond), computing technologies (AI/ML), and data sciences will be leveraged to develop digital health solutions.
- Medical device technology, including point-of-care devices and technologies for remote health monitoring.
- Focused technology incubation programs to translate research into products through start-up ecosystem.

### 1.3.7 Anticipated Outcomes of the Gangwal School of Medical Sciences and Technology

GSMST will be the first of its kind institution in the country with the potential to create an impact on society and economy at local, national and global scale. It is anticipated that the outcome of the School at IIT Kanpur will contribute to overall betterment of existing healthcare.

*Healthcare Service*: The proposed super-speciality hospital along with world-class faculty on board, will offer affordable treatment in super-specialities like oncology, cardiology, nephrology neurology, etc., to over 4 million people in the 300 km radius of Kanpur. Besides, the School would also take-up research in public health issues and help the government in epidemiological survey, forecast and strategic plans using innovative mathematical and computational tools.

*Human Resource Development*: IIT Kanpur, with its well-known brand name in teaching and research, proposes to train and nurture next-generation medical engineers for the country.

*Technology and devices*: Develop affordable devices, technologies, and engineering solutions to unmet medical needs of the country, especially in rural areas.

*Entrepreneurship and knowledge economy*: Serve as the hub for nurturing entrepreneurship through start-ups MedTech domain.

**Acknowledgements** Authors acknowledge Director, IIT Kanpur, GSMST Advisory board members and donors for their continued support.

## References

1. https://www.nmc.org.in/about-nmc/introduction/
2. https://natboard.edu.in/aboutus/
3. Deloitte's 2024 Global health care sector outlook: Navigating transformation
4. WHO global healthcare workforce database. Accessed September 2022
5. Invest India.gov.in May 2020: Digital health in the aftermath of COVID-19
6. Digital transformation in healthcare industry: a survey. https://doi.org/10.1007/978-981-19-2416-3_16

# Emerging Materials in Medicine

# 2

Shreya Mehrotra, Aman Nikhil, Purva Gupta, Sandeep Verma, and Ashok Kumar

**Abstract**

The pursuit of materials in medicine demands a significant balance between scientific innovation, patient compliance and ethical considerations. In the ever-transforming landscape of regenerative medicine and biomedical research, medical materials have evolved from inert supports or functional substitutes to key players in promoting tissue function and regeneration. Furthermore, with a greater interdisciplinary approach, materials research is now all set toward reshaping both clinical medicine and patient outcomes. Through this chapter, we have tried to bring forth some of the cutting-edge materials that have shown tremendous potential toward several clinical applications. These advanced materials are not only bioinspired but also offer structural and functional attributes that address the limitation of the traditional clinical research such as smart materials, drug-eluting materials, wearable technology materials, next-generation hemostats and breathable materials. Discussing the limitations of clinical research and how these materials are a best-fit technology, the need of a synergistic interplay between materials innovation, biocompatibility and associated ethical concerns has been highlighted. The chapter further underscores the envisioned future directions, translational scope and challenges with the growing technology and research in this domain.

**Keywords**

Oxygen-releasing · Nitric oxide · Smart materials · Hemostats · Composite materials · Bone-substitutes

S. Mehrotra · A. Nikhil · P. Gupta · A. Kumar (✉)
Department of Biological Sciences and Bioengineering, Indian Institute of Technology Kanpur, Kanpur, UP, India
e-mail: ashokkum@iitk.ac.in

S. Mehrotra
e-mail: smehrotra@iitk.ac.in

A. Nikhil
e-mail: aman.nikhil921@gmail.com

P. Gupta
e-mail: purva.khirniwal@gmail.com

S. Mehrotra · S. Verma · A. Kumar
Centre for Environmental Science and Engineering, Indian Institute of Technology Kanpur, Kanpur, UP, India
e-mail: sverma@iitk.ac.in

S. Verma
Department of Chemistry, Indian Institute of Technology Kanpur, Kanpur, UP, India

S. Verma · A. Kumar
Centre of Excellence for Materials in Medicine, Gangwal School of Medical Sciences and Technology, Indian Institute of Technology Kanpur, Kanpur, UP, India

Center for Nanosciences, Indian Institute of Technology Kanpur, Kanpur, UP, India

A. Kumar
The Mehta Family Centre for Engineering in Medicine, Indian Institute of Technology Kanpur, Kanpur, UP, India



S. Verma (ed.), *Technology and Innovation in Medical Sciences*, IITK Directions 7,
https://doi.org/10.1007/978-981-96-8606-3_2

## 2.1 Introduction

The field of medicine and healthcare are seeing phenomenal transformations that are fueled by the innovative advancements in materials science. From serving as a mere-support structure and/or drug-delivery vehicles, today, medical materials/ biomaterials are required to offer a huge range of responsibilities such as reinstate tissue function, aid in tissue transplant, enable in-situ monitoring, provide localized drug delivery, facilitate organ reconstruction, and fully-degrade within the host tissue after fulfilling their designated role [1–3]. Moreover, advanced materials are expected not only to enhance the performance of the medical devices/implants, but also augment several biological functions when used in contact with the patient tissues and organs. This is mainly due to the advent of *avant-garde* technologies that have now enabled the in-depth understanding of the material-cell interactions, the bio-mechanics of materials at cellular interface, and the impact of molecular design, intrinsic material properties, and their three-dimensional hierarchical assembly on cellular functions and tissue re-organization [3]. It has now been well-verified that on varying the material properties such as their mechanical behavior, chemical composition, and structural characteristics at various length scales, a resulting difference can be observed in their biological properties [3–5]. Modulation in these properties can therefore act as potential cues for instructing and directing several biological processes [6–8].

The global medical materials market is valued at $45.2 billion in 2024 and is projected to grow at the CAGR of 7.3%. This includes various materials that are used as therapeutics, wound healing materials and dressings, hemostats, implantable devices and prosthetics, orthopedic and dental implants, materials for cardiovascular and plastic surgeries. Moreover, a great thrust is on devising innovative materials that are sustainable and display high-performance. Some of the key players that are the true drivers of medical material innovations include; (a) improved patient outcomes (b) development of personalized treatment regimens (c) improved diagnosis and (d) ease of disease management [9]. The need for advanced next-generation materials for early and improved diagnosis as well as improved clinical outcomes can be easily understood. For instance, the need of new generation cardiac stents that can allow arterial repair, bioactive materials for enhanced tissue regeneration and healing, development of immuno-isolated devices, next generation pace-makers etc. However, bringing the patients as an equivalent stake holder in innovation strategies can be a little complex. In the present scenario, the healthcare system regards patients as '*experts in their own conditions*' and therefore looks forward to innovations that can either be patient-specific and/ or involve them and their family caregivers as active participants in care [9, 10]. This would require, incorporating materials or developing newer materials for wearable/IoT integration, stimuli-responsive materials or bioinspired materials. Moreover, these materials are also required to add value in the form of improved efficiency, efficacy, quality, sustainability, safety and/ or affordability.

With the aim of developing some of the cutting-edge materials for healthcare, the Center of excellence (CoE) for '*Materials in Medicine*' at the Gangwal School of Medical Science and Technology, Indian Institute of Technology Kanpur focuses on driving innovations that can cater to the present clinical needs. The CoE encompasses of several teams comprising of scientists (with interdisciplinary backgrounds in material science, chemical science, chemistry, biological sciences and polymer sciences), young researchers, clinicians and industrial partners that work together toward developing translational medical materials and products. Through this article, we have aimed at providing a bird's eye view to some of the latest material technologies that have been developed at the CoE, and which offer simple solutions to some of the most complex clinical problems. A few of the outstanding research contributions that are discussed in detail include the development of advanced hemostat materials, oxygen releasing wound dressing materials for diabetic patients, smart polymers for neural regeneration, bioactive bone implants, and anti-bacterial bone cements.

## 2.2 Design and Development of New-Generation Materials for Healthcare

The current needs of the medical science have challenged the material scientist to include the development of implantable biosensors, artificial muscles, bioactive wound dressings, new-generation of drug-eluting implants, bio-adhesives, sealants, multifunctional stents, modern imaging materials, bio-resorbable bone implants and immune-isolation devices. However, many of these needs cannot be met by depending on a single or a simple blend of natural and synthetic materials [11]. Therefore, a paradigm shift can be seen toward developing engineered materials which drive their inspiration from the biological processes. These engineered materials can be described as either natural or synthetic materials that have been chemically/physically/biologically manipulated to offer properties that can be specific to their medical applications, thus enhancing efficacy and improving clinical outcomes [12]. For instance, engineering electrically conductive materials that can enhance the function of muscle and neural tissues, anti-bacterial surface coating materials for preventing post-surgical infections in implants, engineered catechol-based bio-adhesives for improved fistula repair, devising smart pH-responsive materials as targeted cancer treatment modalities and so on. The research teams at IIT Kanpur are pursuing some of the cutting-edge innovations in terms of medical materials. Some of the emerging next-generation materials that have been developed through our research endeavors are described below:

### 2.2.1 Oxygen-Releasing Antioxidant Biomaterials

Oxygen-releasing biomaterials have emerged as a promising innovation in healthcare, especially in tissue engineering where these materials address the critical issue of hypoxia in both the engineered tissues and in the host tissue microenvironment. Hypoxia, a condition characterized by insufficient oxygen supply, can have severe detrimental effects on cellular viability and function, particularly in highly oxygen-dependent cells like pancreatic β-cells, neural cells and cardiomyocytes [13, 14]. In hypoxic conditions, most cells experience impaired functionality and increased oxidative stress, which can further exacerbate cellular damage by generating free radicals that react with proteins and DNA, leading to cellular dysfunction and death [15]. A critical issue that is often noted with biomaterial-based matrices and scaffolds is the poor vascularization within engineered scaffolds or tissues both in vitro conditions as well as during the initial stages of implantation. This issue delays the infiltration of host vasculature, which is crucial for a continuous oxygen supply, thereby prolonging the hypoxic state and hindering tissue regeneration [16].

To overcome these challenges, there is a need for designing oxygen-releasing materials that can mimic the natural oxygen supply in the tissues through the sustained and controlled release of molecular oxygen. Some of the common oxygen-generating compounds, such as sodium percarbonate, calcium peroxide, magnesium peroxide, and hydrogen peroxide, release oxygen through chemical decomposition when exposed to water. However, a significant challenge of using these compounds is the uncontrolled release rate of oxygen. Innovations are required in the design of biomaterials that can not only conjugate or encapsulate these oxygen-releasing compounds but also effectively control the release rate of oxygen. For if not controlled, rapid oxygen release can lead to oxidative damage and the production of free radicals. On similar lines, incorporating antioxidants, such as catalase, can help mitigate free radical damage and could also be an interesting strategy. However, many mixed notions exist regarding the requirement of an over-complicated scaffold design and ensuring enzyme stability [15, 16].

To address these limitations, we have proposed the use of solid peroxides embedded in antioxidant hydrophobic polymers to create scaffolds that release oxygen in a sustained manner while reducing the effects of free radicals. This approach has the potential to reduce tissue necrosis under ischemic conditions, particularly in high oxygen demand cells such as cardiac cells and neurons. Enhancing oxygen availability in scaffolds or matrix materials is crucial during the initial period before host vasculature infiltrates the scaffold, a process that can take one to two weeks. For instance, the use of cryogelation technology has ensured the formation of large, interconnected pores within 3D cellular matrices, facilitating effective oxygen and nutrient diffusion. In one study, the incorporation of calcium peroxide (CPO) into antioxidant polyurethane (PUAO) scaffolds resulted in a sustained release of oxygen over a period of 10 days [15]. The hydrophobic nature of PUAO slowed the diffusion of water, thereby prolonging the release of oxygen. The PUAO-CPO cryogels were effective in preventing necrosis in an in vivo skin flap model, while the PUAO antioxidant scaffold alone delayed the onset of necrosis (Fig. 2.1a) [15]. These findings suggest that the oxygen-releasing capability of PUAO-CPO scaffolds significantly contributes to tissue preservation under ischemic conditions and has potential applications in next-generation tissue engineering strategies.

Oxygen-releasing antioxidant scaffolds have also been studied in complex disease conditions associated with ischemia, such as chronic diabetic wounds and myocardial infarction. Chronic diabetic wounds represent a significant health issue, often leading to high rates of amputation due to impaired healing processes characterized by hypoxia and oxidative stress. A novel wound dressing, OxOBand, was developed by combining an oxygen-releasing antioxidant scaffold with exosomes derived from adipose-derived stem cells (ADSCs) [16]. This innovative dressing enhanced the healing process in keratinocytes and fibroblasts under hyperglycemic and oxidative stress conditions (Fig. 2.1b). In vivo studies using a diabetic rat model revealed that the OxOBand significantly accelerated wound closure rates, re-epithelialization, and granulation tissue formation compared to control groups [16]. The treatment reduced inflammation prevented ulceration in infected diabetic wounds, and promoted collagen deposition and maturation, which are essential for healthy skin regeneration.

For cardiac applications, such as myocardial infarction, the use of a bilayered patch consisting of PUAO-CPO and collagen has demonstrated enhanced cardiac function and angiogenesis (Fig. 2.1c) [17]. By delivering sustained oxygen and attenuating oxidative stress, this patch mimics the natural oxygen supply and promotes regeneration. The addition of antioxidant properties helps mitigate the adverse effects of reactive oxygen species (ROS), which are often elevated in hypoxic environments. Moreover, the integration of exosomes with these oxygen-releasing scaffolds further enhances their regenerative potential by

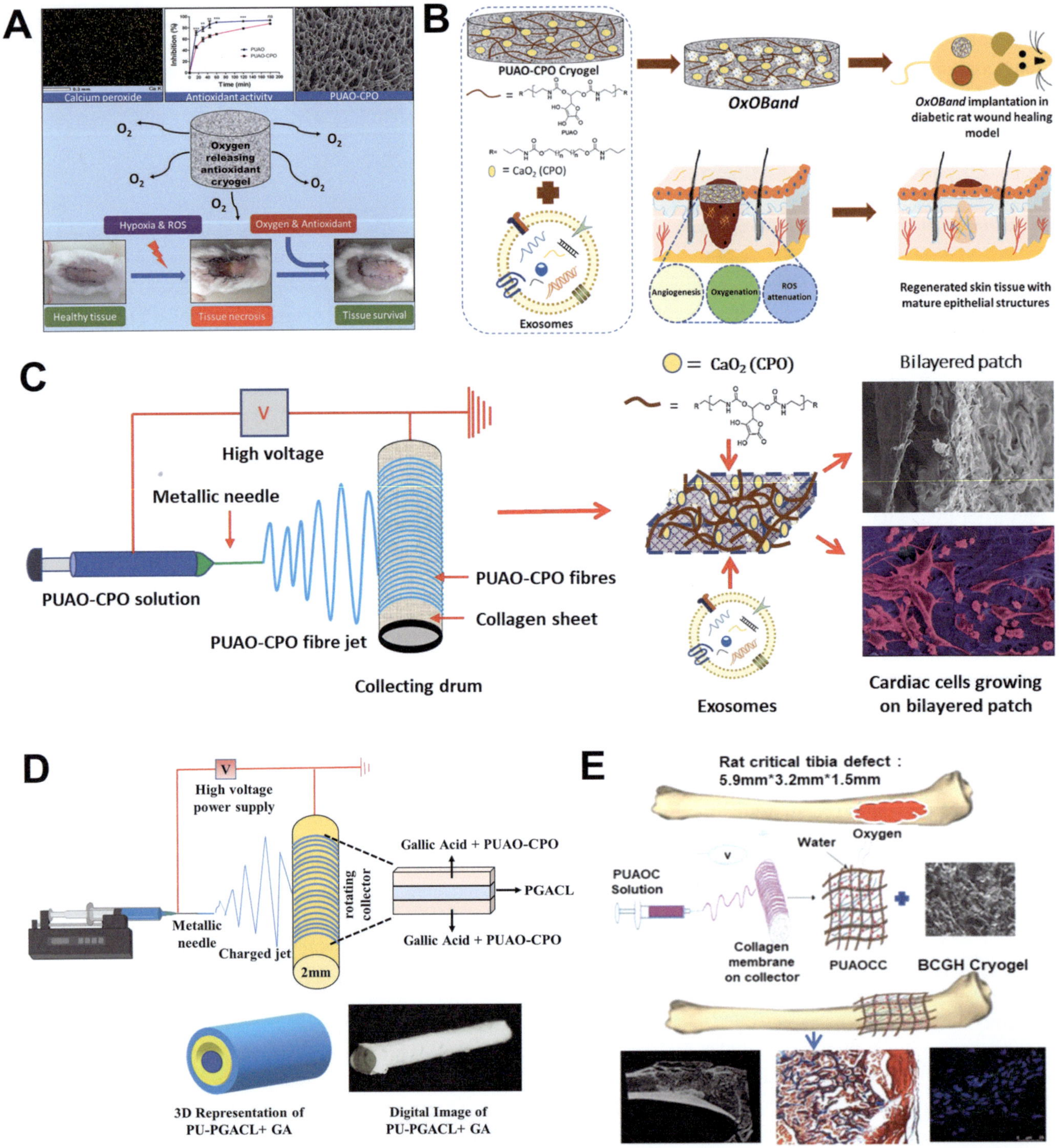


**Fig. 2.1** Design and development of oxygen-releasing materials for various clinical applications. **a** Schematic representation of the oxygen-releasing antioxidant cryogel (PUAO-CPO) along with its properties and application in in vivo ischemic skin flap mode. Reprinted with permission from [15]. Copyright © 2018, American Chemical Society. **b** Schematic representation of the formation of OxOBand from PUAO-CPO with adipose-derived stem cells exosomes for enhancing diabetic wound healing process. Reproduced with permission from [16]. Copyright 2020 © 2020 Elsevier Ltd. **c** Schematic representation demonstrating the development bi-layered cardiac patch for cardiac regeneration after myocardial infarction. Reproduced with permission from [17]. Copyright 2021 © 2021 Elsevier B.V. All rights reserved. **d** Schematic representation of the electrospinning process for fabricating trilayered architecture of the vascular stent. Reproduced with permission from [18]. Copyright 2020 @ 2020 Elsevier Ltd. All rights reserved. **e** Schematic representation of the fabrication of dual-layered PUAOCC membrane to promote the periosteal and bone regeneration in a critical bone defect. Reprinted with permission from [19]. Copyright © 2021, American Chemical Society.

providing additional pro-survival and pro-angiogenic signals, which are vital for tissue repair and regeneration [17]. These results suggest that the combination of antioxidant properties, oxygen release, and exosome-mediated effects can effectively address the multifaceted challenges of diabetic wound healing.

Furthermore, we have also delved into fabricating an oxygen-releasing gallic acid-based vascular graft which successfully addressed the pressing issue of atherosclerosis, a leading cause of cardiovascular disease [18]. Our research focused on incorporating a natural antioxidant, gallic acid, within biodegradable polymers like polycaprolactone (PCL) and polyglycolic acid (PGA) to fabricate an electrospun biomimetic drug-eluting stent (Fig. 2.1d). This vascular stent exhibited dual functionality: supporting the growth and proliferation of endothelial cells while inhibiting smooth muscle cell growth. This is essential for repairing the endothelium lining and promoting vascularization within engineered tissues [18]. These oxygen-releasing multifaceted biomaterials present a promising alternative for cardiovascular disease treatment by addressing existing limitations such as restenosis and adverse immune reactions.

Oxygen-releasing materials have also shown significant promise in enhancing bone healing processes, particularly in challenging environments like large bone defects where hypoxia is a major barrier. The periosteum, a vital component of bone, plays a crucial role in nourishing cortical bone and housing osteoprogenitor cells essential for bone repair. Damage to the periosteum, often resulting from traumatic injuries or surgical interventions, can lead to delayed bone healing and an increased risk of non-union fractures. To mitigate these challenges, bioengineered periosteal substitutes have been developed, composed of electrospun oxygen-releasing antioxidant polyurethane on a collagen membrane (PUAOCC) [19]. This innovative material not only supported primary periosteal cell survival under oxidative stress conditions but also significantly improved bone formation and periosteal regeneration when used in conjunction with a bioactive inorganic–organic composite cryogel (BCGH) in a critical-sized rat tibial bone defect model (Fig. 2.1e) [19]. The sustained release of oxygen from materials like calcium peroxide, incorporated into these substitutes, played a pivotal role in maintaining redox balance. This balance is essential for suppressing oxidative stress, which can otherwise lead to osteoblast and osteocyte apoptosis, enhanced osteoclastogenesis, and ultimately accelerated bone resorption. The gradual and sustained release of oxygen ensured a continuous supply over an extended period, providing a conducive environment for bone regeneration. Additionally, ascorbic acid, a component of PUAOCC, contributes to the antioxidant potential, regulating reactive oxygen species and playing a vital role in collagen synthesis and trabecular bone formation by overexpressing bone matrix genes in osteoblasts [19]. These findings underscore the effectiveness of oxygen-releasing materials in enhancing bone healing by not only providing a sustained oxygen supply but also by mimicking the natural bone repair process, thereby facilitating improved outcomes in bone regeneration therapies.

In summary, oxygen-releasing biomaterials offer a compelling approach to tissue engineering by effectively mimicking the natural oxygen supply, providing a controlled and sustained release of oxygen, reducing oxidative stress, and supporting the physiological processes necessary for tissue healing and regeneration. These materials hold significant potential across a wide range of applications, including chronic wounds, cardiovascular disease, and bone regeneration, marking a significant advancement in the field of regenerative medicine.

### 2.2.2 Nitric Oxide Releasing Biomaterials

Nitric oxide (NO) is a versatile signaling molecule that plays a crucial role in numerous physiological processes, including wound healing, angiogenesis, and vasodilation, making it a valuable agent in promoting tissue regeneration and healing. Its ability to modulate inflammation and immune responses further highlights its potential in regenerative medicine, where it can significantly enhance therapeutic outcomes [20]. NO's capacity to improve blood flow and oxygen delivery to tissues is particularly beneficial for patients recovering from surgical procedures or those suffering from chronic wounds. Additionally, the interplay between NO and other signaling pathways, such as those involving growth factors and cytokines, suggests that combining NO with other therapeutic agents could maximize its benefits in clinical settings. This potential has paved the way for innovative treatment strategies that harness the synergistic effects of NO, leading to more effective interventions in tissue repair and regeneration [21].

Despite its therapeutic promise, a significant research gap exists in achieving controlled and sustained NO release to maximize its benefits while minimizing side effects. Current NO delivery systems often struggle with poor stability and lack of target specificity, which limits their clinical application. Precise modulation of NO concentrations is essential, as its effects vary significantly with concentration and exposure duration [21]. To address these challenges, researchers are focusing on developing novel materials that can respond to physiological stimuli, such as pH or temperature, to enhance targeted NO delivery. This approach ensures that therapeutic levels of NO are maintained at the site of injury while reducing systemic exposure, which is crucial for minimizing potential side effects. Injectable NO-releasing materials, which could provide localized and controlled NO delivery, remain relatively underexplored in biomedical applications [22]. However, recent advancements in polymer chemistry and nanotechnology offer promising prospects for developing innovative formulations that improve the stability and release profiles of these materials, leading to more effective treatments. Integrating these materials with existing drug delivery systems could also create synergistic effects, further enhancing overall therapeutic efficacy and patient outcomes.

Scaffolds enabling sustained NO release offer a promising solution to these challenges by enhancing NO's efficacy in various tissue engineering and regenerative medicine applications while minimizing potential side effects. The integration of advanced imaging techniques could facilitate real-time monitoring of NO release, its effects on cellular responses, and optimal delivery methods, allowing for a more tailored approach to patient care.

A dual delivery system providing antioxidant, and controlled NO-releasing properties has been developed to address the challenges associated with oxidative stress, a common complication in various pathological conditions due to an imbalance in reactive oxygen species (ROS). This system was designed to overcome the limitations of existing NO-releasing materials, such as safety concerns with diazeniumdiolates and short NO release durations, particularly in hydrophilic systems like gelatin. By integrating antioxidants, such as thiols, with the NO-releasing system, researchers created a dual delivery platform that offers sustained and prolonged NO release while maintaining antioxidant action. Specifically, S-nitroso-N-acetyl-L-cysteine (SNAC) was covalently functionalized to gelatin, providing a sustained release of NO alongside antioxidant properties. This dual system not only addresses the interplay between NO and ROS but also offers therapeutic efficacy in tissue engineering applications, potentially benefiting conditions such as chronic wounds and nerve injuries (Fig. 2.2a). The biocompatibility and biodegradability of gelatin make this platform a promising candidate for advanced therapeutic applications, although careful consideration of dosage is necessary to avoid potential toxicity at higher concentrations [20].

The anti-tumorigenic potential of NO-releasing compounds has also been explored through the development of a novel purine derivative designed to ensure sustained NO release at the target site, thereby inducing apoptosis in tumor cells (Fig. 2.2b). NO's involvement in oxidative stress, apoptosis, and regulation of cell cycle progression makes it a useful anticancer adjuvant. However, the gaseous nature and short half-life of NO pose significant challenges for its direct administration to tumor tissues. This has led researchers to explore various NO-donating scaffolds, such as polymeric nanoparticles, dendrimers, and silica nanoparticles, though these have often faced issues related to selectivity, biocompatibility, and safety. To address these challenges, purine derivatives have been investigated due to their crucial role in intracellular signaling pathways. These molecules act as messengers in anti-inflammatory processes and suppression of tumor growth, making them suitable candidates for NO delivery systems. A 6,9-disubstituted purine derivative was designed by functionalizing the C-6 position of the purine ring with a flexible alkyl linker containing an O-$NO_2$ group, allowing controlled NO release following first-order kinetics. This derivative was then used to develop new scaffolds that regulated NO release to ensure safe and effective therapeutic approaches. The scaffold exhibited anti-proliferative, anti-migratory, and anti-clonogenic effects on HepG2 cell lines, indicating its potential against the metastasis of hepatocellular carcinoma (Fig. 2.2b). The observed effects may be due to NO's interactions with inorganic molecules, prosthetic groups, or DNA structures, and its involvement in pathways such as cGMP-dependent or cGMP-independent pathways. Despite its potential, the therapeutic application of NO remains controversial, necessitating extensive studies to further establish its physiological effects and explore combinatorial therapies with nonconventional systems, such as immunotherapy, photodynamic therapy, or photothermal therapy (PTT), to overcome multidrug resistance with NO donor derivatives in future [22].

Combinatorial treatment approaches using NO-releasing compounds are also being explored to combat complex chronic wounds associated with persistent inflammation, oxidative stress, microbial infections, and ischemic conditions. Chronic wound healing requires comprehensive reparative and regenerative solutions that can provide a multifaceted release of growth factors and cytokines necessary to limit the feedback loop of existing trauma and relieve patients from the physical and mental burden. One study addressed this challenge by fabricating an innovative janus bilayer cryogel-based scaffold designed to mimic the skin's ultrastructure, effectively supporting cell proliferation, migration, and antioxidant activity, leading to expedited wound closure in infected chronic wounds within 21 days. This scaffold was developed by incorporating a chitosan–gelatin layer with NO and oxygen ($O_2$)-releasing particles, cerium oxide ($CeO_2$) for antioxidative properties, and a polyvinylpyrrolidone-iodine (PVP-I) layer for antibacterial action (Fig. 2.3a). The 3D cryogel matrix is particularly effective for developing wound dressings due to its porous structure, which allows for nutrient and oxygen exchange, high exudate absorption, and tunable mechanical properties. The fabricated scaffold demonstrated reduced necrosis and preserved normal skin ultrastructure in an ischemic wound rat model, showcasing the effectiveness of NO and $O_2$ releasing properties (Fig. 2.3b). Histological analysis revealed healthy skin ultrastructure with granular tissue, blood vessels, and collagen deposition, while the presence of the CD31 marker indicated angiogenesis with enhanced collagen I expression. These findings suggest that the scaffold is biocompatible and exhibits strong antibacterial action against common pathogens such as *Escherichia coli*

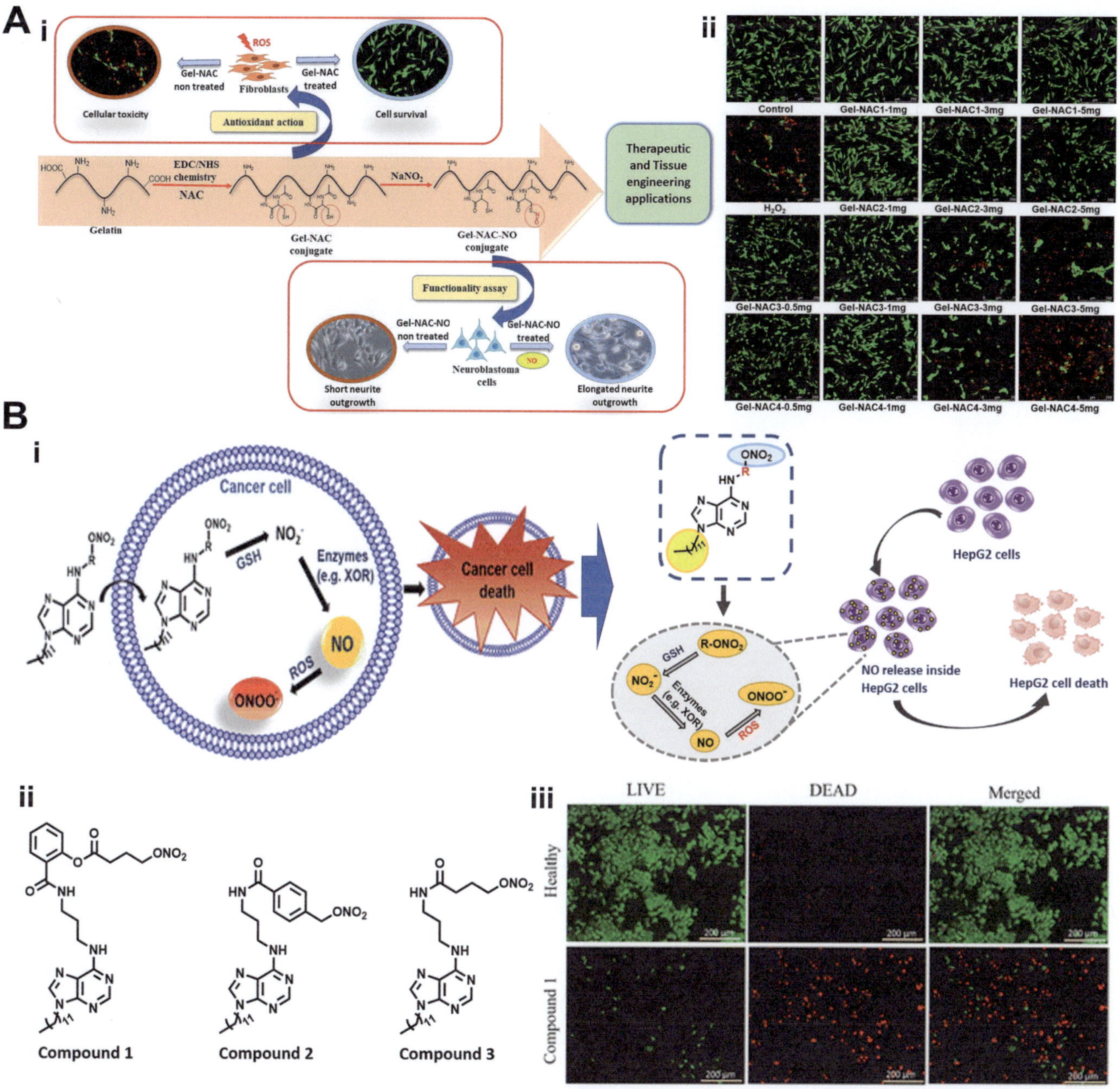


**Fig. 2.2** Design and application of Nitric-oxide releasing materials. **ai** Schematic representation of the preparation of the Gel-NAC and Gel-NAC-NO conjugates and their functional efficacy in fibroblasts and neuronal cell line, **aii** Live dead cell assay showing effects of Gel-NAC variants on $H_2O_2$ induced toxicity. Calcein AM (green) staining showing cellular viability after $H_2O_2$ treatment. Whereas PI (red) staining showing cellular death induced by $H_2O_2$ and higher concentration of Gel-NAC conjugates. Reprinted with permission from [20]. Copyright 2021 © 2021 Elsevier Ltd. All rights reserved. **bi** Schematic representation of the plausible NO release mechanism by purine derivatives inside the cells that leads to cell death. GSH = glutathione; ROS = reactive oxygen species; and XOR = xanthine oxidoreductase. **bi** Structures of the different compounds synthesized. **biii** The apoptosis assessment with C-AM/PI after treatment of HepG2 cells with compound 1 as compared to control depicted with fluorescence images at 20 × magnification (Live-C-AM-green; Dead-PI-red). Reproduced with permission from [21]. Copyright 2024 © 2024 Elsevier Ltd. All rights reserved

and *Staphylococcus aureus*, indicating that the combinatorial approach using multifaceted scaffolds is effective for treating complex wound conditions. The developed scaffold, with its prolonged and sustained release profile of NO and $O_2$, could be a promising dressing material for chronic wounds, offering valuable insights into future clinical applications [22].

Furthermore, NO's significant role in various physiological processes, including wound healing and nerve repair, has positioned it as a valuable addition to the domain of 3D printing. The incorporation of NO-like bioactive cues is being explored to

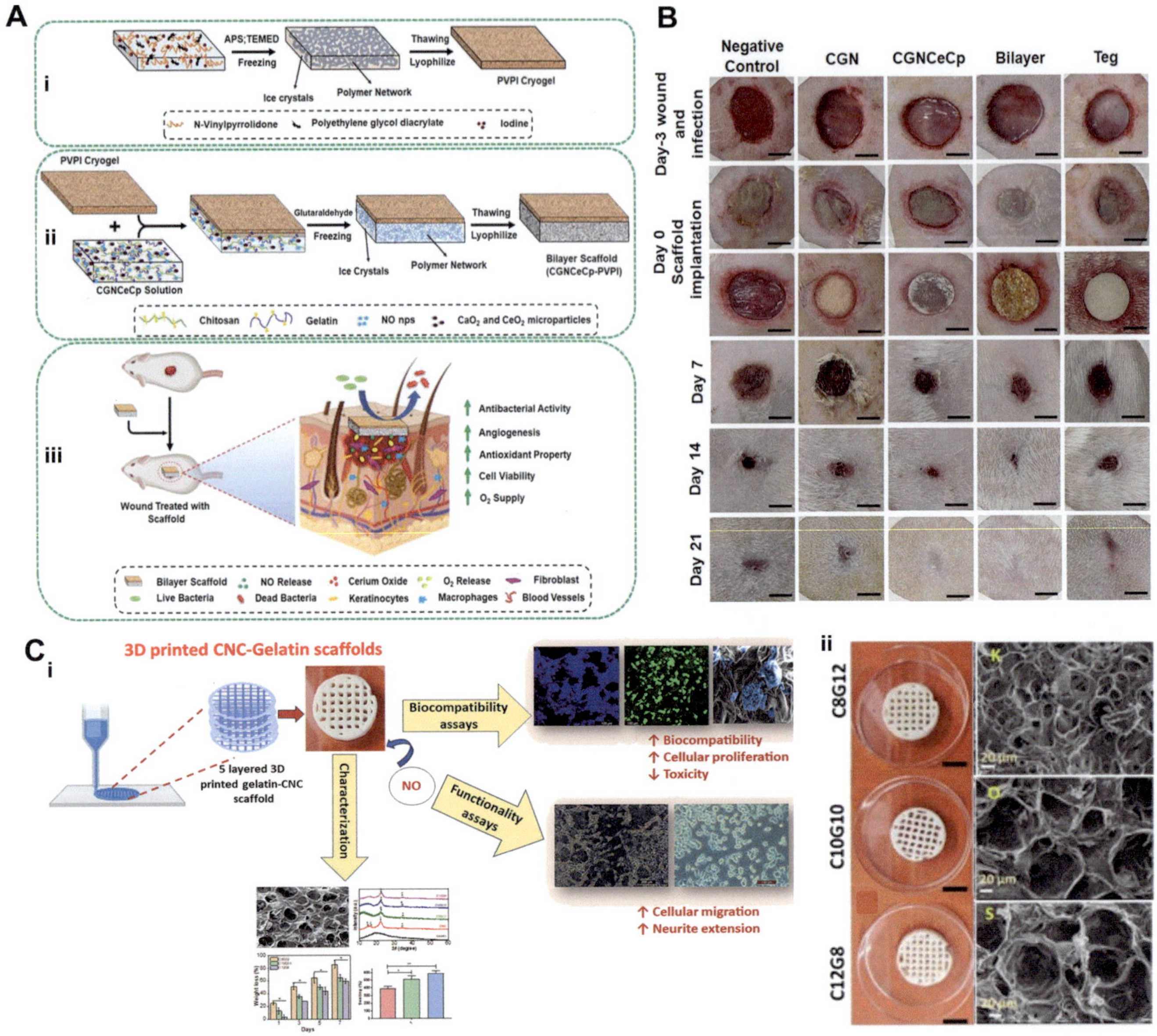


**Fig. 2.3** Materials for delivery of NO and its application in wound healing. **a** Schematic illustration of the overall work (i) synthesis of the PVP-I cryogel layer from precursor polymeric solutions, (ii) synthesis of bilayer scaffold (CGNCeCp-PVPI) through cryogelation, (iii) treatment of chronic wounds by implantation of the synthesized scaffold. Reprinted with permission from [22]. Copyright 2023 © 2023 Elsevier B.V. All rights reserved. **b** Representative digital images of the infected chronic wound, implanted scaffolds and healing progress over a period of 21 days, scale bar: 4 mm, Reprinted with permission from [22]. Copyright 2023 © 2023 Elsevier B.V. All rights reserved. **ci** Schematic representation of the 3D Printed cellulose nanocrystals and gelatin scaffolds with bioactive cues for biomedical applications. **cii** The digital images depict mesh objects printed using the C8G12, C10G10, and C12G8 formulations, respectively (scale bar 15 mm). Reprinted with permission from [23]. Copyright 2024 © 2024 Elsevier B.V. All rights are reserved, including those for text and data mining, AI training, and similar technologies

enhance the regenerative and therapeutic properties of scaffolds. Advances in tissue engineering and regenerative medicine, particularly in developing biocompatible scaffolds that replicate the ultrastructure of biological tissues, have opened new possibilities in organ transplantation, in vitro drug testing, and the creation of biomimetic platforms. Unlike traditional fabrication techniques such as hydrogelation, freeze-drying, and electrospinning, 3D-printed scaffolds offer structural precision, controlled parameters, and reproducibility. The precision at the ultrastructural level and the ability to incorporate bioactive cues make these scaffolds highly suitable for tissue engineering applications, including skin, bone, and cartilage repair and regeneration. For example, 3D-printed cellulose nanocrystal (CNC) hydrogels have been explored in combination with modified gelatin functionalized with NO (Fig. 2.3c). The functionalization process involves surface coating the 3D-printed scaffolds with NO-modified gelatin, enabling sustained NO release. The CNC hydrogels impart unique properties to the 3D-printed scaffolds, such as biodegradability, mechanical strength, swelling capacity, biocompatibility, and flexibility toward surface modifications. Functionality assays, such as scratch and neurite outgrowth tests, demonstrated the positive effects of NO on cell migration and neurite length, further validating the approach. This innovative method of incorporating NO into 3D-printed scaffolds represents a novel approach in the field, combining the advantages of 3D printing with the therapeutic benefits of bioactive cues, thus opening new avenues for advanced biomedical applications [23].

### 2.2.3 Smart-Materials or Stimuli-Responsive Materials

Smart materials, also known as stimuli-responsive materials, have immense potential in the healthcare domain. These materials usually undergo reversible changes in their physical or chemical properties in response to external stimuli like temperature, pH, light, magnetic or electric fields, and mechanical stresses [24]. These can be utilized in targeted therapeutic or drug delivery applications at the site and often become crucial materials of choice for minimally invasive surgical applications. Some of the well-known smart polymers include poly(N-isopropyl acrylamide) (PNIPAAm), poly(N-vinyl caprolactam) (PNVCL), and pluronics which are now being increasingly utilized in regenerative medicine.

In a recent study, we have reported the use of a bioactive thermoresponsive smart polymer poly(N-vinyl caprolactam) (PNVCL) loaded with clot-busting exosomes (derived from HT1080, a human fibrosarcoma cell line) for its application in clot lysis and as a clinical solution for treating thrombosis [25]. The material was synthesized using free radical polymerization and showed the lower critical solution temperature (LCST) behavior at 31 °C. It meant that below LCST the material is in liquid form and above the LCST it forms a gel (Fig. 2.4ai). This thermo-responsive property was utilized for targeted delivery of the exosomes. For therapeutic purposes, PNVCL was used to encapsulate HT1080 exosomes, which has urokinase rich molecular cargo. Role of HT1080 exosomes in treating whole blood clot was also established in vitro (Fig. 2.4aii). Pre-clinical evaluation of this therapeutic intervention was performed in rat carotid artery model for treatment of thrombosis (Fig. 2.4aiii) [25]. Streptokinase encapsulated inside PNVCL, used as experimental control, was also tested for its delivery at the clot site. The ultrasound imaging confirmed that our material-based intervention was able to dissolve the blot clot and hence resulted in increased diameter of the occluded vessels. Histological analysis confirmed that our bioactive thermo-responsive material-based therapeutic intervention was able to restore the intimal organization of the vessel similar to the healthy tissue, thus stating the efficacy of these materials in treating thrombosis.

Another thermoresponsive formulation that was developed, found its application in mucosal healing of the inflamed gut tissue [26]. A topical therapy was developed by conjugating temperature-responsive polymer PNIPAAm with hyaluronic acid to make a sprayable therapeutic formulation with LCST of 35 °C (Fig. 2.4bi). The formulation has the property to adhere to damaged gut mucosa because of its temperature-induced phase transition and mucoadhesive properties. A ex vivo adhesion experiment established the mucoadhesive properties of this formulation by depicting the formation of a thin physical coating of the therapeutic formulation on the mucosal lining at a physiological temperature within 5 min (Fig. 2.4bii). Physicochemical characterization of (P(NIPAM-co-NTBAM)-HA) established this formulation to be biocompatible, hemo-compatible, and non-immunogenic. A perfusion-based microphysiological device was designed to culture rat colon explants and study the potential of the formulation in mucosal healing and regeneration (Fig. 2.4biii). Prednisolone (a steroid based drug) was encapsulated within the thermos-responsive PNIPAAm-HA polymer formulation to achieve maximum therapeutic efficacy in the case of inflammatory bowel disease-like conditions. This was assessed using rat colon explants cultured in the custom-fabricated perfusion-based micro-physiological device. Histological analysis suggests that the prednisolone-encapsulated polymer formulation restored the mucosal architecture after 2,4,6-trinitrobenzenesulfonic acid-induced damage to a great extent (Fig. 2.4biv). The results also justified the potential of clinical translation because of its targeted delivery, ease of customization, long shelf life, and minimal side effects.

Apart from using stimuli-responsive polymers, innovative strategies also revolve around incorporating conductive nano-materials within the well-established medical polymers. These nano-materials because of their hierarchical structure are able to provide better control over the material properties and often result in enhanced clinical outcomes. One of our endeavors involved the development of a nerve wrap termed “Electroband”, which was fabricated by electrospinning of chitosan, gelatin, and reduced graphene oxide (rGO) (Fig. 2.5a) [27]. This nerve wrap displayed high biocompatibility, biodegradability, cell-instructive and an electrically conductive nature. Pre-clinical studies involved testing these ‘Electrobands’ in median nerve compression and transection injury rat models along with external electrical stimulation and a small dose of nerve growth factor (NGF) (Fig. 2.5b). The goal of the study was to link the utilization of conductive scaffolds with standard electrical stimulation procedures to reduce the clinical translational gaps.

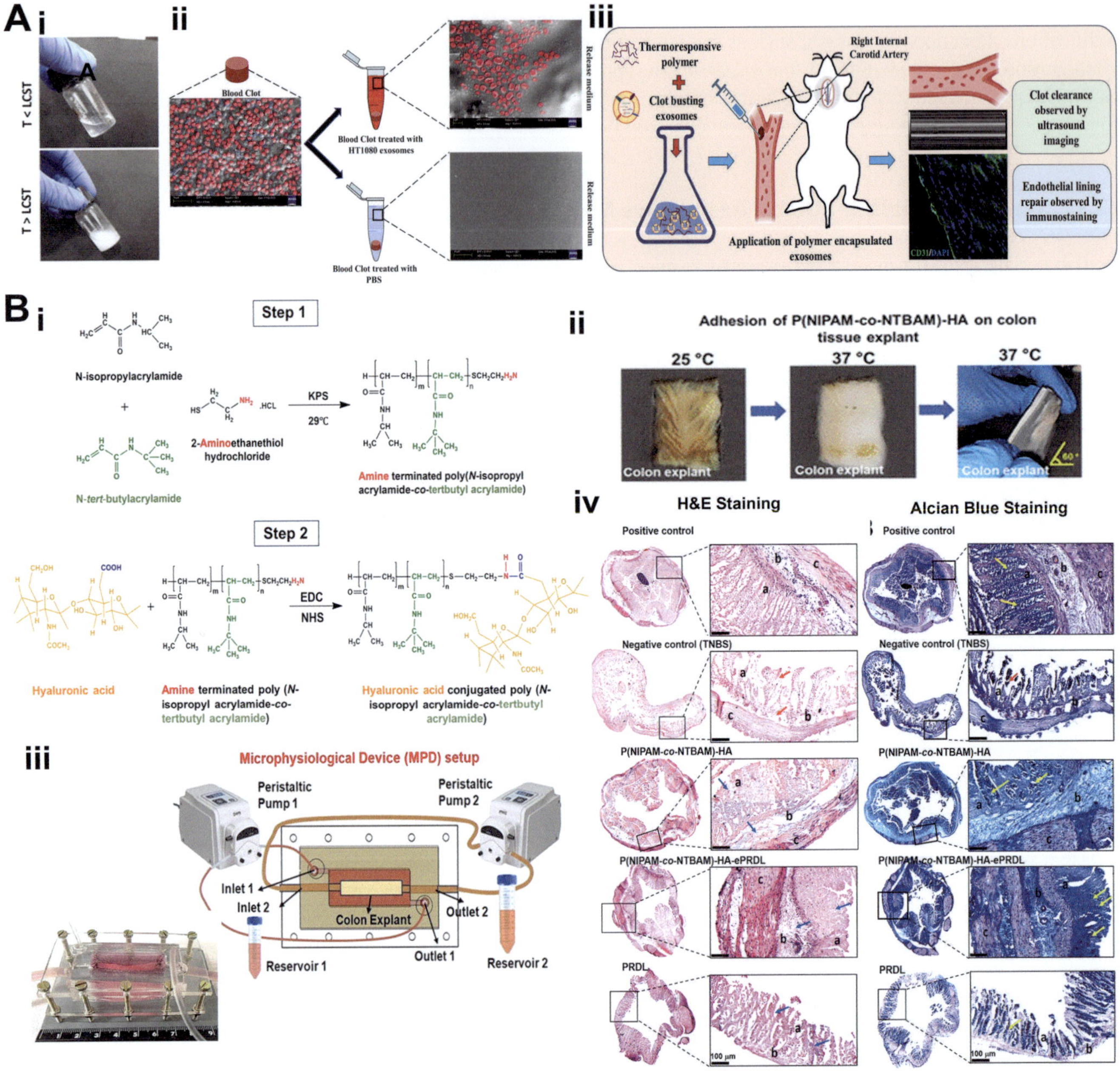


**Fig. 2.4** Stimuli-responsive materials and their immense potential for clinical applications. **a** Use of Poly(N-vinyl caprolactam) (PNVCL) for treating thrombosis. **ai** Digital image showing transition of PNVCL from sol-to-gel at a temperature below and above LCST. Reproduced with permission from [25]. Copyright 2022 © 2022 Published by Elsevier Ltd. **aii** Representative scanning electron micrograph of whole blood clot, scale bar–10 μm; whole blood clot treated with exosomes (20 μg/mL), scale bar–2 μm; and whole blood clot treated with PBS control, scale bar–10 μm at 12 h time point. Reproduced with permission from [25]. Copyright 2022 © 2022 Published by Elsevier Ltd. **aiii** schematic showing the application of PNVCL loaded with HT1080 exosomes in rat carotid artery thrombosis model. **b** A thermo-responsive polymer-based therapy for treating inflammatory bowel disease. **bi** A two-step reaction schematic displaying the formation of amine-terminated poly(N-isopropylacrylamide-co-tert-butyl acrylamide) [P(NIPAM-co-NTBAM)-$NH_2$] in step 1 and hyaluronic acid-conjugated poly(N-isopropylacrylamide-co-tert-butyl acrylamide) [P(NIPAM-co-NTBAM)-HA] in step 2. **bii** Images displaying the mucoadhesive properties of P(NIPAM-co-NTBAM)-HA. A thick adhesive coating of the polymer formulation was seen to form on the colon epithelium beyond LCST temperatures (37 °C) **biii** Schematic showing the perfusion-based microphysiological device setup administration of therapeutic formulations into the lumen of the colon tissue explant and digital image of the bioreactor chamber harboring the rat colon tissue explant. **biv** Histological analysis showing hematoxylin and eosin-stained and alcian blue-stained images of TNBS-damaged rat colon epithelium cultured in a perfusion-based microphysiological device and treated with P(NIPAM-co-NTBAM)-HA, PDRL alone, and P(NIPAM-co-NTBAM)-HA-ePRDL. Reproduced with permission from [26]. Copyright 2022 © 2022 Published by Elsevier Ltd

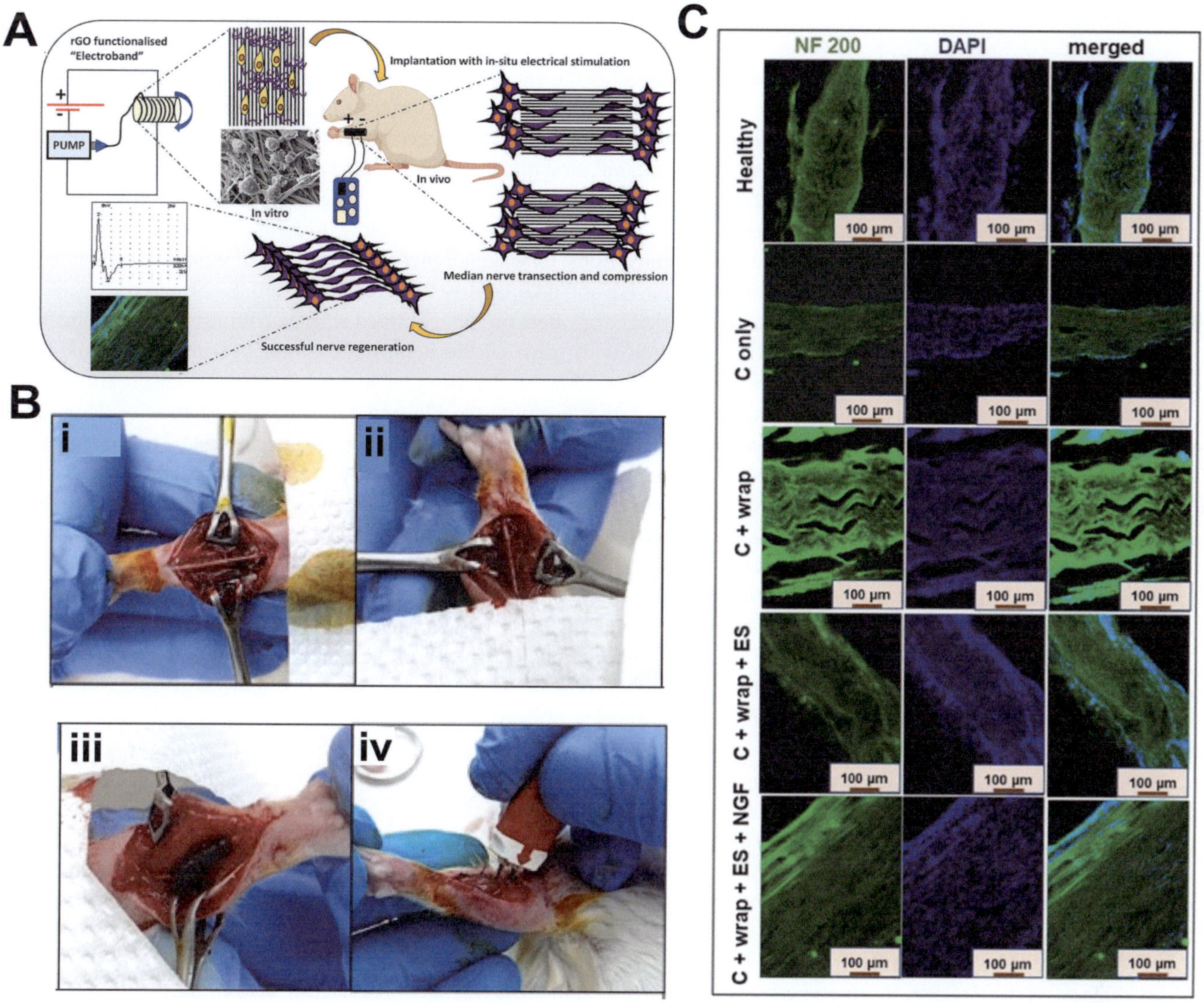


**Fig. 2.5** Incorporating conductive nano-materials for enhancing functional properties of materials. **a** Schematic displaying the fabrication of rGO functionalized electrospun 'Electrobands' for peripheral nerve regeneration. **b** Pictorial representation of surgical procedure depicting. (i) a healthy median nerve after forearm incision and muscles removal. (ii) median nerve after compression of nerve for 30 s resulting into significant disruption of myelin sheath. (iii) "Electroband" wrapped (similar manner for both the injuries) around the compressed nerve. (iv) the scaffold implantation was followed up with intraoperative in-situ electrical stimulation of 3 V, 20 Hz for 10 min continuously. **c** Immunostaining images depicting the growth of compressed nerve fibers with NF 200 demonstrating fascicular arrangement of nerve fibers in healthy control, incomplete regeneration in C only, aligned growth of nerve fibers in C + W underlining the significance of nanofibrous scaffold, fascicular growth of nerve fibers on conjugation of electroactive wrap with electrical stimulation in C + W + ES and exuberant growth of nerve fiber with combinatorial therapy in C + W + ES + NGF. Adapted with permission from [27]. Copyright 2023 © 2023 Published by Elsevier Ltd

The combination of rGO functionalized wrap, electrical stimulation and NGF resulted in enhanced growth of nerve fibers through as well as within the scaffold. This could be assessed with the maximum expression of NF 200 as observed in case of C + wrap + ES + NGF group when compared with the control group (Fig. 2.5c). A promising outcome was seen in terms of peripheral nerve tissue regeneration and reversal of proper fore-limb impulses in rats, thus establishing it as a potential medical material.

### 2.2.4 Advanced Hemostat Materials

The most critical driving factor of the global hemostat market is the surge in the number of world-wide surgical procedures, civilian and defense blood loss traumatic cases. They have provided impetus to give a strong boost to the rising incidence of bleeding complications during surgeries, accidents and military actions. This necessitates the development of advanced and high-quality hemostat products that promote faster blood coagulation and healing effects without any introduction of surgery-associated infections. Various hemostatic products fabricated using polymers (chitosan, gelatin, cellulose, collagen, fibrin sealant and cyanoacrylates), zeolites and smectite are already commercially available worldwide. However, technological gaps still exist leaving a large scope for material-based innovations. One such drawback is the lack of wound size adaptability (most commercially available bandages are insufficient in size and adaptability to cover deep, stellate, or massive incisions). The materials, especially those present in the Indian market, work best on flat, confined surfaces, limiting their applicability in extreme scenarios. Another drawback that is associated with some of the hemostatic products (such as granule-based hemostats-Quickclot) is the leaching of material/medicinal residues in the vascular lumen. As a result, distal arterial flow is likewise blocked by these medications. Some hemostats that promote the clotting pathway can potentially damage the endothelium and spread clots intraluminally, leading to distal thrombosis. Hemostatic agents also provide a risk of infection. Slow clotting of blood, toxicity, mechanical durability, expenses, non-antiseptic, and allergic reactions are the main downsides of these dressings. Therefore, there is a need of smart and shape memory dressing material that efficiently controls blood coagulation at injury site as well as synergistically promote would healing and regeneration without any side effects.

In this scenario, we have been successful in developing a hemostatic prototype (CryoHaemoClot-bandages) which displays superior material and biological properties in comparison to the commercially available products in the Indian market when assessed on a laboratory scale and pre-clinical animal experiments (TRL 4). The developed and patented hemostatic prototype (CryoHaemoClot-bandages) comprises of chitosan and functionalized-dextran incorporating kaolin and calcium ($Ca^{2+}$) (hemostatic agents) all of which have been put together in a product using the cryogelation technology (Fig. 2.6) [28]. The addition of aldehyde groups to biodegradable dextran resulted in improved coagulation and promoted crosslinking without the use of hazardous chemicals thus making it a simple and easily adaptable technology for the clinical setting (Fig. 2.6a). The interconnected pore structure of the cryogel imparts it an excellent shape memory ability and can therefore be employed for use in various hemorrhagic wounds (Fig. 2.6b). The prototype when assessed for its blood clotting efficiency in comparison to Axiostat and Quikclot® displayed faster blood clotting, sustained clot formation, and strong antibacterial action (Fig. 2.6c). In vitro analysis displayed significant decrease in clotting time (~30 s); higher platelet/red blood cell aggregation; improved wound healing capacity, and activation and good bacterial growth inhibition (E. coli and S. aureus). It could further be elucidated that the developed CryoHaemoClot activated both intrinsic and extrinsic coagulation pathways, by reducing aPTT and PT by ~ 58% and 31%, respectively.

The efficacy of the developed prototype (CryoHaemoClot-bandages) was also assessed in vivo in non-compressible rat liver and femur hemorrhagic models, where it performed significantly better in preventing blood loss and reducing clotting time at the injury site in comparison to clinically used Axiostat and Quikclot®. Further, the mechanical stability, flexibility, and shape memory ability supported in its usage to stop uncontrolled bleeding even at irregular, non-compressible wounds. Initial TRL4 results have shown that the developed CryoHaemoClot can work as a significantly improved technology for bleeding control applications; and therefore, future endeavors are now directed toward development of this product as per national/international industrial and clinical standards.

### 2.2.5 Functionalized Composite Bone Substitutes

Bone injuries are one of the most critical injuries when a person suffers from trauma or fractures arising due to any metabolic disorders. Although allografts are considered the gold standard, donor site morbidity and their limited availability has become a challenge in clinical scenarios [29]. In such cases, bone graft substitutes become suitable alternatives for the treatment of bone defects. These are extensively characterized by advanced techniques to elucidate their properties and decide their suitability as bone substitutes for biomedical applications. Our research endeavors have resulted in the formulation of an indigenously bone nanocement (NC), consisting of nano-hydroxyapatite (nHAP) and calcium sulfate (CS) in a 60:40 ratio, that forms an injectable paste and has the property to set in 15 min [29]. This serves as a clinically feasible option for the surgical intervention for filling bone defect voids. nHAP constitutes a natural component of the bone while CS resorb in a few months leading to the formation of a porous structure assisting in osteoconduction [29]. This nanocement can also be functionalized with bioactive factors to make it osteoinductive and enhance overall bone regeneration. In one of the studies, the delivery of bioactive factors

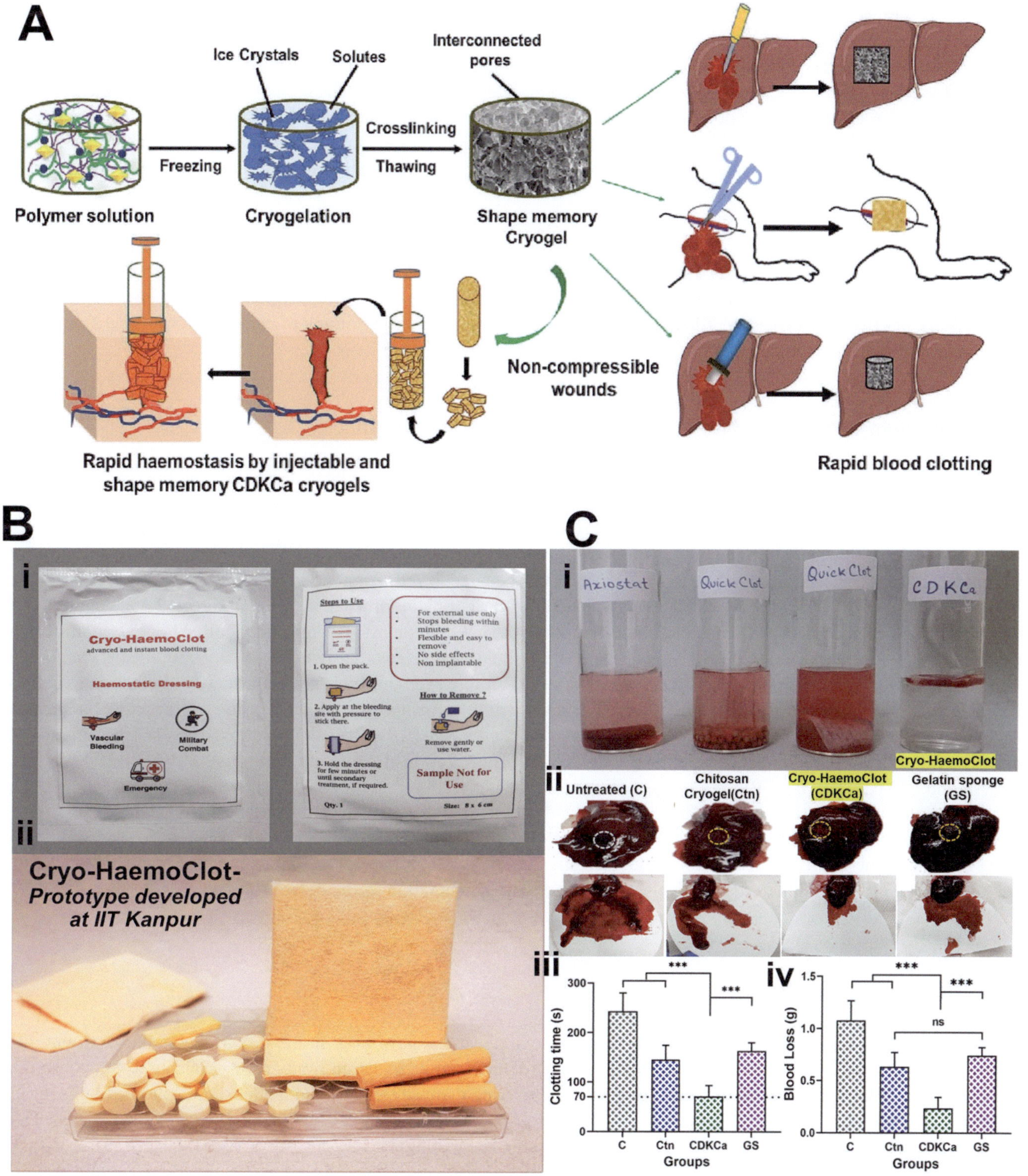


**Fig. 2.6** Venturing into advanced hemostat materials. **a** Schematic showing fabrication of cryogel scaffold (consisting of chitosan, functionalized dextran, with hemostatic agents like kaolin and calcium) with its different applications in blood clotting and **b** Representation of the developed prototype (CryoHaemoClot-bandages) at IIT Kanpur and its ability to be fabricated in various formats depending on wound depth and size. **c** The developed prototype (CryoHaemoClot-bandages) displays superior blood absorption, blood clotting efficiency, and reduce clotting time in comparison to commercially available Axiostat and QuikClot® hemostats. Adapted with permission from [28]. Copyright 2023 © 2023 Published by Elsevier Ltd

like bone recombinant human morphogenetic protein 2 (rhBMP-2) and zoledronic acid (ZA) in cranial bone defect using this nanocement were investigated. Micro-Computed Topography (μ-CT) and histological assessment revealed regeneration in NC + rhBMP-2 + ZA group in comparison to empty, NC-only, NC + ZA and empty groups (Fig. 2.7a) [29]. This NC was also tested in an osteoporotic and osteomyelitis-induced bone fracture [30], where the combination of bone marrow-derived mesenchymal stem cells (bMSCs) along with BMP-2, ZA, and rifampicin (antibiotic) were loaded in NC resulted in bone regeneration in the fracture site and the bone formed was mechanically strong and free from infection (Fig. 2.7b). NC has extensive application as an injectable filler in bone defects where it can be applied with ease of applicability, even when functionalized with several bioactive factors.

Recent advancements have been carried out in developing organic–inorganic polypropylene fumarate (PPF) and nanohydroxyapatite (nHAP) based composites which were utilized as carriers of antibiotics for treating osteomyelitis [31]. The in vivo rat subcutaneous model showed that this biomaterial has reduced the bacterial burden completely at the infected site and aided in the enhancement of bone regeneration in dead spaces created during surgical debridement after an injury. Further, work has been performed in utilizing PPF with PCL and nHAP for 3D printing of construct for critical size injuries at load-bearing sites in the goat model.

### 2.2.6 Polymer-Composite Materials for Bone Tissue Regeneration

Cryogels often find their application in bone tissue engineering, where nHAP has been utilized in combination with natural polymers like gelatin and chondroitin sulfate to make a composite macroporous cryogel scaffold, for subchondral bone of the osteochondral tissue [32]. Briefly, the cryogel has nHAP particles embedded in the pore walls with a good interconnected pore network that allowed the proliferation of pre-osteoblasts. This cryogel has later been applied in animal models, where bone regeneration in the subchondral region of the knee has been achieved. Another, cryogel-based scaffold consisting of collagen, gelatin, and nHAP was fabricated and then loaded with rifampicin for its application in infected bone injuries [33]. This antibiotic-loaded cryogel prevented biofilm formation in the in vitro conditions while augmenting bone formation in the defect site when functionalized with BMP-2 and ZA in the animal model. Treating critical-size bone injuries is challenging and the limitations associated with the clinical use of autografts require synthetic bone grafts that can be designed in a patient-specific fashion using printing that provides control over architecture, porosity, and rigidity. The use of composite photocuring resin made up of poly(trimethylene carbonate) (PTMC) with ceramic [nHAP or tri-calcium phosphate (TCP)] were utilized to make a 3D printed scaffold using stereolithography (SLA) (Fig. 2.7ci) [34]. Different scaffolds PTMC (P), PTMC-nHAP (P-HA), and PTMC-TCP (P-TCP) were imaged using scanning electron microscopy which showed the intricate architecture of the 3D printed scaffolds (Fig. 2.7cii). These scaffolds were then impregnated with cryogel made up of gelatin-ceramic to fill the pores of the cryogel and then functionalized using BMP-2 and ZA as per optimized dosages to enhance the osteoinductivity of the scaffolds. The fabricated scaffold was then investigated in the rabbit bone defect model and the results indicated that these functionalized scaffolds have effectively carried out bone regeneration in the defect site and showed the potential of SLA fabricated scaffolds as patient-specific next-generation bone substitute grafts (Fig. 2.7ciii and civ).

### 2.2.7 Bioresorbable Alloys

Bioresorbable alloys especially magnesium-based for bone applications have been in the research domain for a long time due to their mechanical properties and osteoconduction but their rapid degradation limits their application. So, controlling the degradation is the key to improving their properties and making them suitable for biomedical applications. In this regard, efforts have been made to purify magnesium using a melt self-purification approach and then reinforcing using 0.6% nHAP and 0.6% strontium substituted nHAP [35]. To control their rate of degradation, a low-cost stir-assisted squeeze casting method was employed. These magnesium-based alloys were extensively characterized and for animal testing, small cylindrical pins with 2.7 mm diameter and 2 mm height were fabricated and implanted in rat femur shaft critical size bone defect. The results showed osteoconduction and new bone formation along the side of implanted magnesium pins with a controlled degradation profile, thereby showing their potential application for orthopedic implant fixtures.

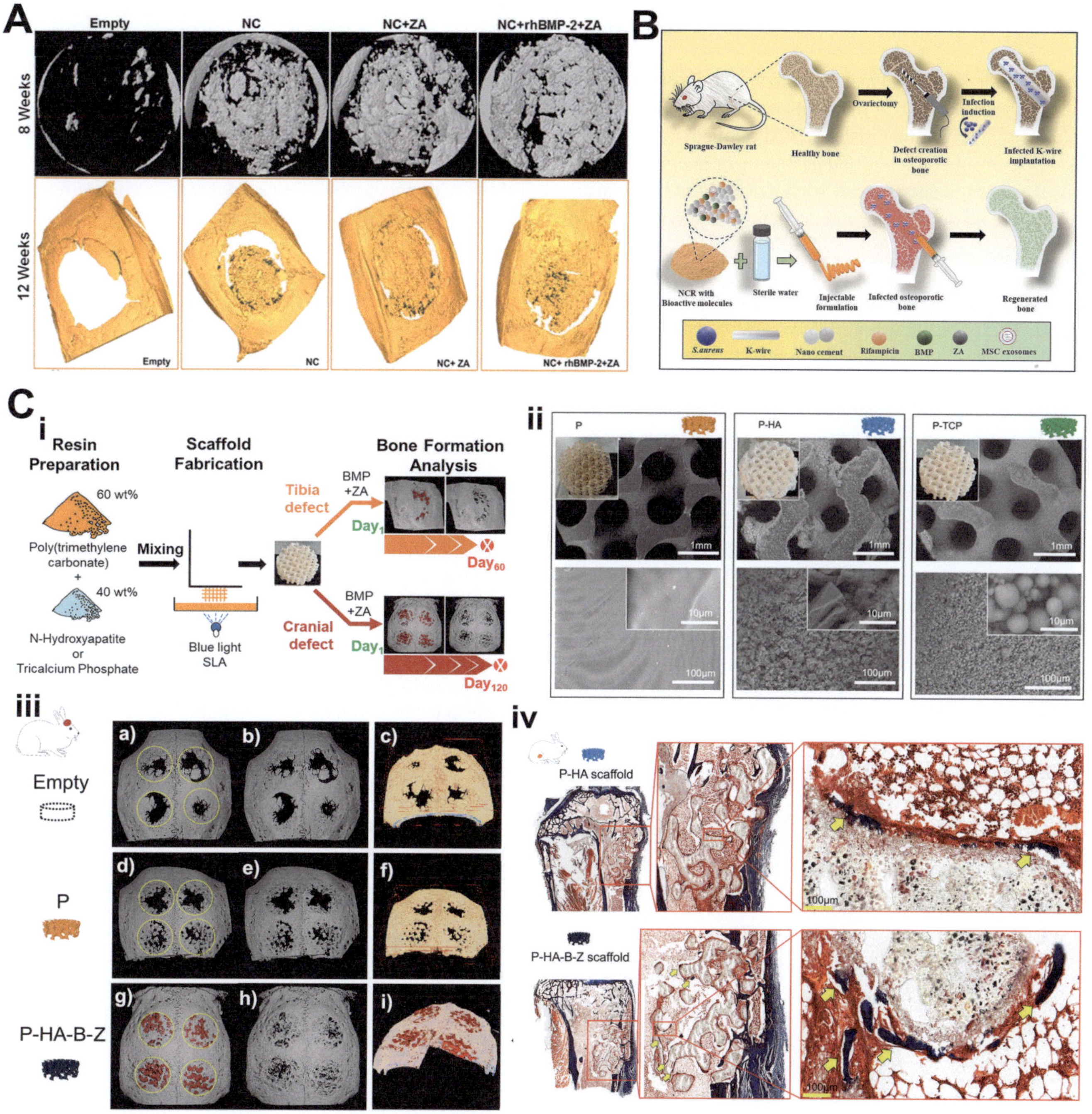


**Fig. 2.7** Establishing bioactive materials for bone tissue engineering applications. **a** Micro-CT images showing surface rendered 3D model images of defect site at 8 week and micro-CT rendered image of defect site at 12-week time point displaying the amount of highly mineralized volume present at the defect and bone material integration. Reproduced with permission from [29]. Copyright 2017 © 2017, American Chemical Society. **b** Schematic showing the application of nanocement loaded with BMP-2, ZA, and rifampicin in osteoporosis and osteomyelitis-induced bone fracture. **ci** Schematic displaying formulation of photocuring composite resins with poly(trimethylene carbonate) containing high ratios of bioactive ceramics and printed porous 3D composite scaffolds to be used as bone grafts. **cii** SEM images displaying the structural and surface characterization of scaffolds. **ciii** Micro-CT 3D rendered images representing defect margins (yellow circles) and implanted scaffolds in three groups. The scaffolds are visualized in red or have been removed by thresholding to show tissue mineralization. **civ** Masson's Trichrome staining analysis of bone tissue formation in tibia defects. Yellow arrows mark the infiltrated osteoblasts and mineralized tissue deposited on the scaffold surface. The scaffold provides a conductive surface for cell infiltration and bone formation at the interior parts of the defect at independent sites. Reproduced with permission from [34]. Copyright 2020 © 2020, American Chemical Society

## 2.3 Existing Challenges and Future Directions

It is well understood that materials do have a great impact on the healthcare system just as they have on the on the pharmaceuticals. A large number of materials ranging from metals and alloys, ceramics, composites, polymers, nanomaterials to now biologically derived materials are finding their specific applications in the clinical setting. Therefore, great efforts need to be made in carefully selecting and designing of materials. This should preferably be done in close consultation with the clinicians as well as the industry experts such that it eases the translation of these materials to the clinics. Most of the current research that focuses on developing and designing new synthetic materials show great material properties but are greatly imperfect in their biomedical application. One of the ways in which this can be prevented is that while developing new materials systems, the researchers should start by associating the materials with patient needs rather than looking for solutions off the shelf. It is believed that when catering to the patient needs, will drive the motivation for new material designs that can cater to issues such as quality of life, performance, safety, risk of failure, lifespan, and replacement strategies.

Most of the future directions in this domain are towards developing smart materials, cell-instructive materials, wearable materials, and bio-active materials which can cater to patient needs and care. With the advent of state-of art technologies such as 3D Printing, Computer Numerical Control (CNC) machining, Electromechanical robotics, Artificial Intelligence and Machine Learning (AI-ML) approaches, Internet Connected Object (ICO) for IoT platforms, research in this domain is taking all leaps and bounds to reach the forefront of translational science and clinical practice. This reflection can be seen in the form of several patient specific implants, wearable technologies, automated control of palliative care devices, advanced wound care materials, and minimally-invasive micro-injectable materials that are now reaching the markets and are adding a new dimension to medicine. However, a number of other clinical factors should be well considered while working towards translational materials research. These include regulatory and manufacturing constraints (e.g., material complexity, ease of scalability, and batch to batch reproducibility), material corrosion, consistency in material performance, and its biocompatibility and biodegradability over time [36]. Translational challenges are known to greatly impact the commercial success of any newly developed material in medicine. A common denominator for all types of translational materials, that are moving towards commercialization and translation, is a controllable and reproducible manufacturing process [37]. Even though a huge scope of taking materials in medicine towards clinical translation exist, it is equally important that the emerging 'think' materials should be able to answer all questions pertaining to scalability, manufacturability, reproducibility, compatibility, patient safety and sustainable performance.

**Acknowledgements** The authors would like to acknowledge the funding received from Ministry of Education (MoE STARS, India), Indian National Academy of Engineering (INAE), Department of Science and Technology (DST), Govt. of India, Science and Engineering Research Board (SERB), Indian Council of Medical Research (ICMR), and Department of Biotechnology (DBT), Govt. of India for various projects under which the research work has been carried out. The authors would also like to acknowledge Gangwal School of Medical Sciences and Technology, IIT Kanpur for their funding and support. S.M. acknowledges the Department of Science and Technology, Govt. of India for the Inspire faculty financial support.

## References


1. Morais JM, Papadimitrakopoulos F, Burgess DJ (2010) Biomaterials/tissue interactions: possible solutions to overcome foreign body response. AAPS J 12(2):188–196
2. Zhang YS, Khademhosseini A (2017) Advances in engineering hydrogels. Science (New York, N.Y.) 356(6337)
3. Othman Z, Cillero Pastor B, van Rijt S, Habibovic P (2018) Understanding interactions between biomaterials and biological systems using proteomics. Biomaterials 167:191–204
4. Battiston KG, Cheung JWC, Jain D, Santerre JP (2014) Biomaterials in co-culture systems: towards optimizing tissue integration and cell signaling within scaffolds. Biomaterials 35(15):4465–4476
5. Mehrotra S, de Melo BAG, Miscuglio M, Kiaee K, Shin SR, Mandal BB (2022) Mimicking native heart tissue physiology and pathology in silk fibroin constructs through a perfusion-based dynamic mechanical stimulation microdevice 11(6):2101678
6. Vermeulen S, Tahmasebi Birgani Z, Habibovic P (2022) Biomaterial-induced pathway modulation for bone regeneration. Biomaterials 283:121431
7. Blache U, Ford EM, Ha B, Rijns L, Chaudhuri O, Dankers PYW, Kloxin AM, Snedeker JG, Gentleman E (2022) Engineered hydrogels for mechanobiology. Nat Rev Methods Prim 2:98
8. Park H-J, Hong H, Thangam R, Song M-G, Kim J-E, Jo E-H, Jang Y-J, Choi W-H, Lee M-Y, Kang H, Lee K-B (2022) Static and dynamic biomaterial engineering for cell modulation 12(8):1377
9. Reinius M, Mazzocato P, Riggare S, Bylund A, Jansson H, Øvretveit J, Savage C, Wannheden C, Hasson H (2022) Patient-driven innovations reported in peer-reviewed journals: a scoping review. BMJ Open 12(1):e053735

10. Engle RL, Mohr DC, Holmes SK, Seibert MN, Afable M, Leyson J, Meterko M (2021) Evidence-based practice and patient-centered care: doing both well. Health Care Manage Rev 46(3):174–184
11. Council NR (2001) Materials in the new millennium: responding to society's needs. The National Academies Press, Washington, DC
12. Introduction: bioinspired and biomimetic materials (2017). Chem Rev 117(20):12581–12583
13. Zhao Y, Xiong W, Li C, Zhao R, Lu H, Song S, Zhou Y, Hu Y, Shi B, Ge J (2023) Hypoxia-induced signaling in the cardiovascular system: pathogenesis and therapeutic targets. Signal Transduct Target Ther 8(1):431
14. Tsuyama T, Sato Y, Yoshizawa T, Matsuoka T, Yamagata K (2023) Hypoxia causes pancreatic β-cell dysfunction and impairs insulin secretion by activating the transcriptional repressor BHLHE40 24(8):e56227
15. Shiekh PA, Singh A, Kumar A (2018) Oxygen-releasing antioxidant cryogel scaffolds with sustained oxygen delivery for tissue engineering applications. ACS Appl Mater Interfaces 10(22):18458–18469
16. Shiekh PA, Singh A, Kumar A (2020) Exosome laden oxygen releasing antioxidant and antibacterial cryogel wound dressing OxOBand alleviate diabetic and infectious wound healing. Biomaterials 249:120020
17. Ahmad Shiekh P, Anwar Mohammed S, Gupta S, Das A, Meghwani H, Kumar Maulik S, Kumar Banerjee S, Kumar A (2022) Oxygen releasing and antioxidant breathing cardiac patch delivering exosomes promotes heart repair after myocardial infarction. Chem Eng J 428:132490
18. Das A, Ahmad Shiekh P, Kumar A (2021) A coaxially structured trilayered gallic acid-based antioxidant vascular graft for treating coronary artery disease. Eur Polym J 143:110203
19. Gupta S, Teotia AK, Qayoom I, Shiekh PA, Andrabi SM, Kumar A (2021) Periosteum-mimicking tissue-engineered composite for treating periosteum damage in critical-sized bone defects. Biomacromol 22(8):3237–3250
20. Singh P, Prasad A, Andrabi SM, Kumar A (2021) Synthesis, characterization and in vitro evaluation of a gelatin-based platform with antioxidant and nitric oxide releasing property. Eur Polymer J 150:110395
21. Bormon R, Srivastava E, Ali R, Singh P, Kumar A, Verma S (2024) Anti-proliferative,-migratory and-clonogenic effects of long-lasting nitric oxide release in HepG2 cells. Chem Commun 60(26):3527–3530
22. Singh P, Andrabi SM, Tariq U, Gupta S, Shaikh S, Kumar A (2023) Functionally multifaceted scaffolds delivering bioactive compounds for treatment of infectious chronic and ischemic wounds. Chem Eng J 457:141359
23. Singh P, Baniasadi H, Gupta S, Ghosh R, Shaikh S, Seppälä J, Kumar A (2024) 3D-printed cellulose nanocrystals and gelatin scaffolds with bioactive cues for regenerative medicine: Advancing biomedical applications. Int J Biol Macromol 278:134402
24. Mehrotra S, Dey S, Sachdeva K, Mohanty S, Mandal BB (2023) Recent advances in tailoring stimuli-responsive hybrid scaffolds for cardiac tissue engineering and allied applications. J Mater Chem B 11(43):10297–10331
25. Das A, Nikhil A, Kumar A (2022) Preparation of thermo-responsive polymer encapsulated exosomes and its role as a therapeutic agent for blood clot lysis. Colloids SurfS B, Biointerfaces 216:112580
26. Mairal A, Mehrotra S, Kumar A, Maiwal R, Marsal J, Kumar A (2024) Hyaluronic acid-conjugated thermoresponsive polymer-based bioformulation enhanced wound healing and gut barrier repair of a TNBS-induced colitis injury ex vivo model in a dynamic perfusion device. ACS Appl Mater Interfaces 16(5):5382–5400
27. Srivastava E, Qayoom I, Singh A, Kumar A (2023) A reduced graphene oxide functionalized electrospun nerve wrap: amalgamating electrical and biochemical cues to enhance nerve regeneration in median nerve injury model. Carbon 213:118226
28. Andrabi SM, Kumar A (2023) A kaolin/calcium incorporated shape memory and antimicrobial chitosan-dextran based cryogel as an efficient haemostatic dressing for uncontrolled hemorrhagic wounds. Biomater Adv 150:213424
29. Teotia AK, Raina DB, Singh C, Sinha N, Isaksson H, Tägil M, Lidgren L, Kumar A (2017) Nano-hydroxyapatite bone substitute functionalized with bone active molecules for enhanced cranial bone regeneration. ACS Appl Mater Interfaces 9(8):6816–6828
30. Nikhil A, Qayoom I, Das A, Kumar A (2024) Preventing septic implant failures in osteoporotic hip fractures using antibiotic-loaded functionalized nanocement. Chem Eng J 486:149908
31. Qayoom I, Prasad A, Srivastava E, Fazili KM, Nussler AK, Kumar A (2024) Organic-inorganic composite of polypropylene fumarate and nanohydroxyapatite as carrier of antibiotics for the treatment of bone infections. Biomater Adv 157:213714
32. Nikhil A, Kumar A (2022) Evaluating potential of tissue-engineered cryogels and chondrocyte derived exosomes in articular cartilage repair. Biotechnol Bioeng 119(2):605–625
33. Qayoom I, Srivastava E, Kumar A (2022) Anti-infective composite cryogel scaffold treats osteomyelitis and augments bone healing in rat femoral condyle. Biomaterials Adv 142:213133
34. Teotia AK, Dienel K, Qayoom I, van Bochove B, Gupta S, Partanen J, Seppälä J, Kumar A (2020) Improved bone regeneration in rabbit bone defects using 3D printed composite scaffolds functionalized with osteoinductive factors. ACS Appl Mater Interfaces 12(43):48340–48356
35. Shaikh S, Qayoom I, Sarvesha R, Kumar A (2023) Bioresorbable magnesium-based alloys containing strontium doped nanohydroxyapatite promotes bone healing in critical sized bone defect in rat femur shaft. J Magnes Alloy 11(1):270–286
36. Kowalski PS, Bhattacharya C, Afewerki S, Langer R (2018) Smart biomaterials: recent advances and future directions. ACS Biomater Sci Eng 4(11):3809–3817
37. Serban MA (2016) Translational biomaterials—the journey from the bench to the market—think 'product.' Curr Opin Biotechnol 40:31–34

# 3 Design and Development of a Minimalistic Slider-Crank Mechanism Based Obstacle Overcoming Wheelchair

Nayan Jyoti Baishya and Bishakh Bhattacharya

**Abstract**

This study presents a wheelchair design that incorporates a slider-crank mechanism to enhance stability while navigating obstacles. Traditional wheelchairs experience significant inclination changes when climbing or descending, which can compromise user safety. To address this issue, the proposed system utilizes a linear actuator to dynamically adjust the chair's inclination, ensuring a more stable ride. The mathematical modelling of the system is based on Newton–Euler equations, which help in analysing its dynamic behaviour. Prototype testing demonstrated the effectiveness of this approach, as the wheelchair successfully overcame obstacles up to 35 mm in height and managed descents from 70 mm elevations with minimal inclination variation. In comparison to conventional wheelchairs, which experienced a $-6°$ inclination shift while descending, the proposed design limited this shift to just 1°, significantly improving comfort and stability. Additionally, the rider remains faced in the direction of motion while climbing or descending, enhancing visibility, safety, and overall confidence. By improving accessibility on uneven terrain, this innovative wheelchair design offers a practical solution for users, reducing discomfort and increasing stability.

**Keywords**

Automated wheelchair · Electric powered · Wheelchair (EPW) · Slider-crank mechanism · Assistive robot · Assistive technologies · Dynamic modelling

## 3.1 Introduction

The strength of our bones and muscles generally deteriorates after a certain age, resulting in partial or complete physical disabilities. Occasionally, physical disabilities may also arise due to some unfortunate accidents or mishaps. The issue has become more threatening with the rapid ageing of the worldwide population [1]. In Japan, the country has the highest proportion of elderly citizens. Between 1980 and 2000, the percentage of the population (above 65), has increased from 9.6 to 17.1% (i.e. an increase of 89%). Furthermore, the proportion of the population aged above 80 has increased by 170%. The percentage of elderly people is being predicted to rise further. According to a survey done in 1996 on physically disabled persons in Japan, more than 3 million people were physically disabled, out of which 1.6 million suffered from motor dysfunction [2]. The situation is not unique to Japan but rather a matter of global concern. Hence, extensive research is being carried out towards the development of assistive devices for elderly and disabled people.

In the field of assistive technologies, many devices have been developed which are quite effective for human commutation. The first wheelchair is reported to be developed in 1783 [3] and since then it has undergone momentous evolution. In the

N. J. Baishya (✉) · B. Bhattacharya
Indian Institute of Technology Kanpur, Kanpur, Uttar Pradesh, India
e-mail: nayanb@iitk.ac.in

B. Bhattacharya
e-mail: bishakh@iitk.ac.in



S. Verma (ed.), *Technology and Innovation in Medical Sciences*, IITK Directions 7,
https://doi.org/10.1007/978-981-96-8606-3_3

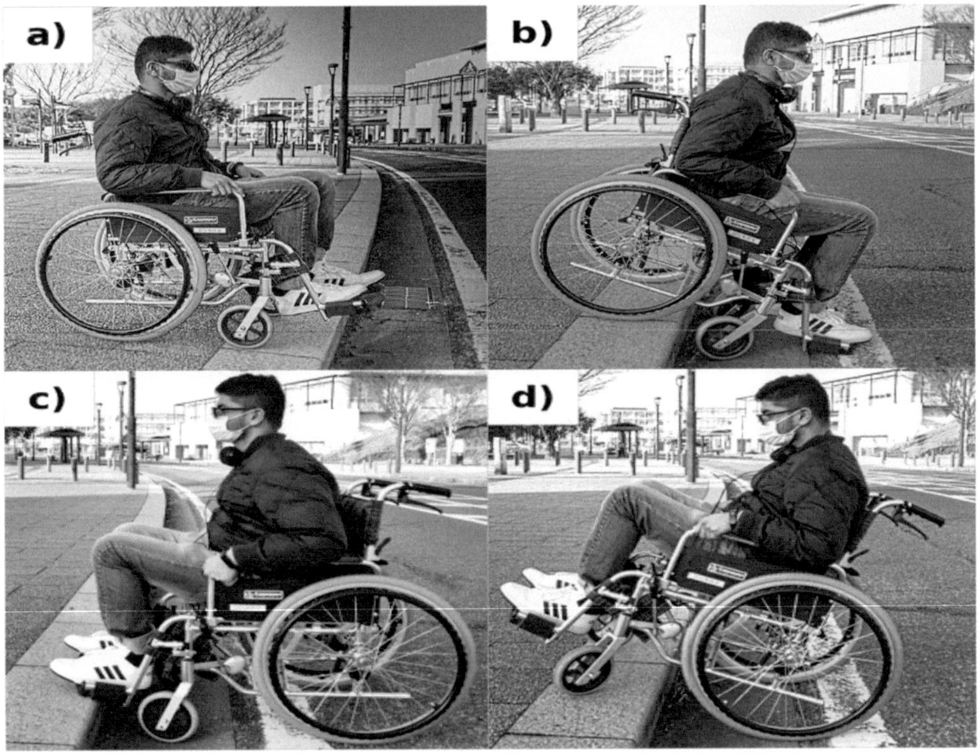


**Fig. 3.1** Variation in inclination angle of the wheelchair while overcoming an obstacle; **a** both front and rear wheels are at elevated platform while descending; **b** front wheels are at lower elevation as compared to rear wheels; **c** both front and rear wheels are at lower platform while ascending; **d** front wheels are at higher elevation as compared to rear wheels

current scenario, electric wheelchairs are being widely used by paraplegic people. Although electric wheelchairs have been very effective, one of the major challenges faced by users is its inability to overcome obstacles.

In Fig. 3.1, the problem faced by wheelchair users, while overcoming an obstacle is shown. Figure 3.1a and b show the situation wherein the rider tries to descend from a higher elevation to lower elevation, while Fig. 3.1c and d describe the situation when the rider tries to ascend from a lower position to higher position. It may be observed from Fig. 3.1b and d that during both ascend and descend, the inclination angle of the wheelchair changes drastically which results in an uncomfortable situation for the rider. Moreover, in some of the cases where the obstacle height is significant, the risk of toppling from the wheelchair may arise.

Significant research has been conducted to develop wheelchairs with climbing capabilities, which can be classified into three main types: tracked systems, articulated leg systems, and hybrid systems. In track-based stair-climbing designs [4–6], track belts are used to propel the wheelchair, allowing it to navigate both stairs and rough terrains effectively. However, these systems tend to be slower in plane than traditional wheel-based designs.

Another approach involves articulated leg mechanisms [7], which enable stair climbing but introduce complex control challenges. To address these limitations, researchers have explored hybrid systems, combining wheels with track belts or wheels with articulated legs [8–10]. These designs allow the wheelchair to switch between different mechanisms, optimizing movement on flat surfaces and steps separately.

Additionally, a modular stair-climbing attachment has been developed [11], which can be connected to a standard wheelchair when needed. This module relies on linear actuators to lift the wheelchair upward. Although this solution is lightweight, it requires assistance from another person, making it more suitable for environments where help is available, such as hospitals or offices.

Studies in [12, 13] have introduced powered linkage-based mechanisms, which incorporate both links and clustered wheels. While the powered links assist in propelling the wheelchair, the clustered wheels facilitate obstacle avoidance. Another innovative approach involves a hybrid system, extensively discussed in a series of articles [14–19], where sliders are utilized to overcome obstacles. In this design, clamps are fixed onto the steps, and sliders then lift the wheelchair [20]. Since the clamps securely grip the stair edges, the risk of slipping during ascent is eliminated. Additionally, this mechanism helps in maintaining the seat's posture while climbing.

Further advancements include wheelchairs capable of both stair climbing and balancing on two wheels [21, 22]. This system employs a pair of wheels on each side, which rotate about a central axis aligned with the midpoint of the wheel centres, enabling step climbing. Another notable innovation achieves stair climbing through multi-limb rotating structures [23, 24].

Researchers have also explored cluster-based stair-climbing wheelchairs, where each standard wheel is replaced by a set of three wheels arranged in a triangular formation [25–32]. These wheel clusters enhance mobility by smoothly rolling over obstacles. Additionally, a four-wheel omnidirectional wheelchair has been developed, utilizing seat tilting to shift the rider's centre of gravity for stair climbing [33]. Other studies focus on heavy-load transport using gears and linkages [34], while Ariga et al. [35] have analysed the wheel dynamics during obstacle climbing.

Most of the commercially available stair-climbing wheelchairs are capable of overcoming obstacles, however, these wheelchairs have some drawbacks. Although track-based wheelchair is efficient in obstacle overcoming, these are slow in planar motion as compared to wheel-based systems. Moreover, some of these systems can climb only in reversed motion. i.e., the riders cannot look directly in the direction of the motion. This may result in a sense of insecurity to the rider. In articulated leg-based systems, the step climbing is achieved by simultaneously controlling multiple actuators. This requires complex and expensive control algorithms, which results in an increase in the overall cost of the system. Hence, a low-cost obstacle overcoming wheelchair with higher safety measure is a need of the hour. This article proposes a minimalist obstacle-overcoming wheelchair equipped with two motors on the front wheels for planar movement. Additionally, a slider-crank-based actuation mechanism connects the rear wheel to the wheelchair frame, enabling it to overcome obstacles. During ascent or descent, an Inertial Measurement Unit (IMU) sensor detects changes in the wheelchair's inclination angle. According to the sensed variation in the inclination angle of the wheelchair, the controller proportionally triggers the linear actuator of the slider crank mechanism. The rear wheel of the wheelchair is attached to the front frame (which is connected to the front wheels) by means of the proposed slider crank mechanism. Any change in length of the linear actuator results in varying the centre distance between the rear and front wheel, thus reducing any variation in the inclination angle of the wheelchair. The proposed system comprises a simple mechanism with fewer actuators which accounts for allow cost of development. The initial development of the proposed mechanism can be referenced from the published articles [36–38]. Use of slider-crank mechanism to achieve obstacle climbing is also proposed by Mori et al. [39]. In this research, at first the front caster wheels are raised by tilting the wheelchair (with external assistance or advanced wheelchair riding skills) and then slider-crank mechanism is used to raise the middle wheels. In this article, the inclination angle of the wheelchair is continuously sensed and slider-crank mechanism is used to minimize the variation in inclination angle of the wheelchair. The following sections discuss the details of the proposed mechanism and the experimental results.

This manuscript is structured as follows: Sect. 3.2 explains the working principle, while Sect. 3.3 covers the design parameters and system modelling. Section 3.4 provides a brief overview of the developed wheelchair prototype. Section 3.5 presents the experimental results, and finally, Sect. 3.6 concludes the study.

## 3.2 Working Principle

In what follows is the working methodology of the proposed mechanism for obstacle overcoming wheelchair. Figure 3.2a and b show the schematic illustrating ascending scenario, whereas Fig. 3.2c and d describe descending scenario. In the proposed wheelchair, for overcoming obstacle, three wheels are used, i.e., two as front wheels and one as rear wheel. The two front wheels are attached to either side of the front frame. The rear wheel is linked to the front frame through a fixed link and a linear actuator.

Figure 3.2a and c represent the configuration of the wheelchair where both the links connecting the rear wheel to the frame of the wheelchair are rigid links, whereas Fig. 3.2b and d show that one of the two links is replaced by a linear actuator. Varying the length of a linear actuator, the distance between the centre of the rear and front wheels may be altered. This in turn minimizes the variation in inclination angle of the wheelchair during ascend and descend over an obstacle. It may be noticed that changing the length of the linear actuator will force the other rigid link to rotate with respect to the joint connecting the link to the frame of the wheelchair. This rigid link is termed as 'crank' and the link representing the linear actuator is termed as 'connecting link'. Such an arrangement where three links are connected in a way, where varying the length of one link results in rotation of the other link or vice-versa, is known as a slider-crank mechanism.

It is important to note that if the wheelchair is built with rigid links, as illustrated in Fig. 3.2a and c, its inclination angle ($\theta$) will fluctuate based on the elevation changes of the front and rear wheels. During ascent, $\theta$ will increase, while during descent, it will decrease accordingly. In some cases, depending on the wheelchair's design and the stair configuration, the inclination angle might become negative, leading to a risk of toppling. To prevent such instability, the inclination angle must

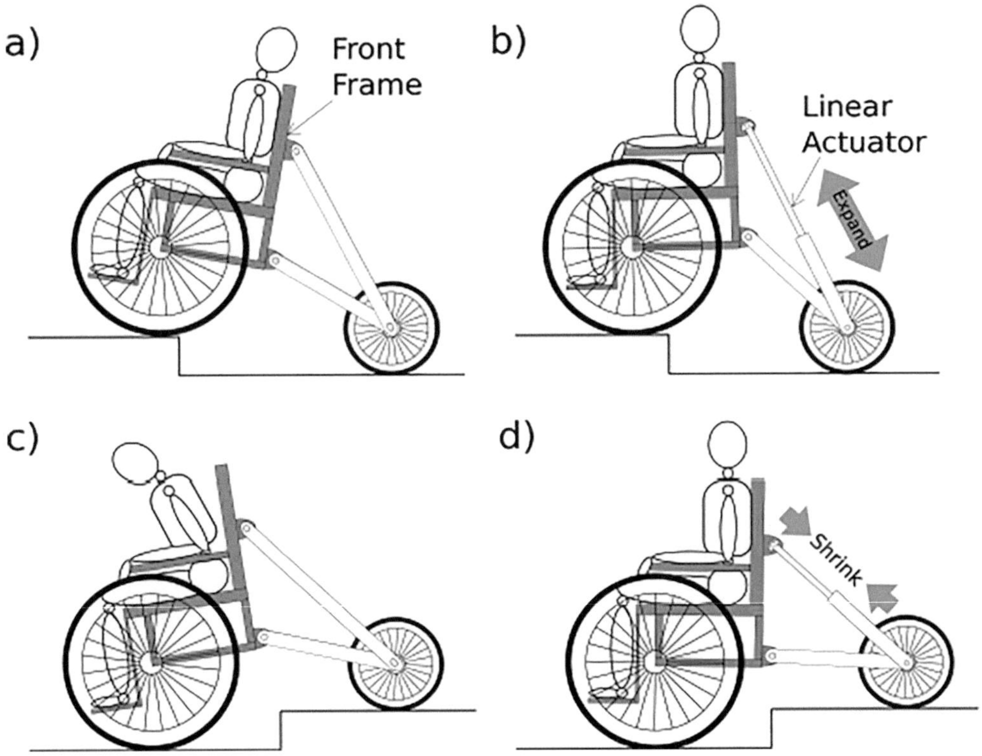


**Fig. 3.2** Schematic demonstrating working principle of the proposed wheelchair; **a** while ascending with rigid links; **b** while ascending with proposed mechanism; **c** while descending with rigid links; **d** while descending with proposed mechanism

be dynamically controlled. This is achieved by adjusting the length of the linear actuator, which connects the rear wheel to the wheelchair frame.

An IMU (Inertial Measurement Unit) continuously monitors any changes in the wheelchair's inclination angle while traversing obstacles. The detected signals are transmitted to a controller, which then regulates the linear actuator's length. As a result, fluctuations in the inclination angle are minimized, enhancing stability and safety. The following section provides a detailed discussion on the design and system modelling of the proposed wheelchair.

## 3.3 Design and System Modelling

In this section, the development of a mathematical model of the proposed system is discussed. This model analyses the kinematic and dynamic behaviour of the wheelchair during obstacle climbing. Additionally, mathematical equations are derived to determine the operating range of the linear actuator, which controls the variation in inclination angle, ensuring the wheelchair's safe operation while overcoming obstacles.

### 3.3.1 Key Design Parameters

This section outlines the parameters defining the proposed wheelchair. Figure 3.3a presents a schematic representation of the design. Relation between $d$ and $\theta$ of wheelchair in plane is shown in Eq. 3.1. However, if the front and rear wheels are at different elevations, $R$ and $r$ in Eq. 3.1 are replaced by elevation of the centre of the front and rear wheels, respectively.

$R$ Front wheel radius
$r$ Rear wheel radius
$L_{cr}$ Length of Crank
$d$ Horizontal projection of $L_{cr}$
$L_a$ Length of linear actuator (connecting link)
$H_c$ Distance between joint C and D

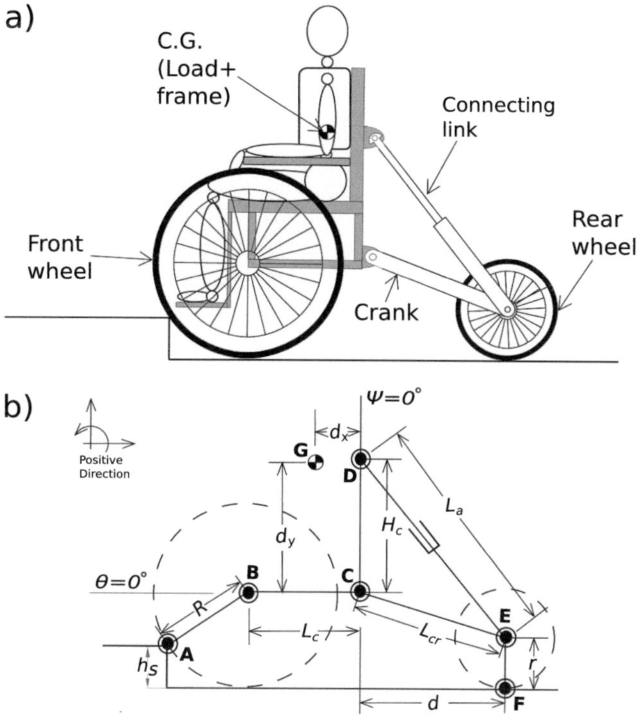


**Fig. 3.3** **a** Schematic of wheelchair with slider-crank mechanism; **b** link wise representation of proposed wheelchair (front and rear wheels are considered as a link)

$L_c$ Distance between joint B and C
$\theta$ Angle of chair with horizontal (Inclination angle)
$\psi$ Tilt angle of link joining joint C and D with respect to the vertical
$d_x$ Horizontal offset of C.G. from point C
$d_y$ Vertical offset of C.G. from seat point C
$h_s$ Height of Obstacle

$$d = \sqrt{L_{\text{cr}}^2 + (R + L_c \sin\theta - r)^2} \tag{3.1}$$

$$L_a = \sqrt{\begin{array}{c}(d - H_c \sin(\theta + \psi))^2 + \\ \left(\sqrt{L_{\text{cr}}^2 - d^2} + H_c \cos(\theta + \psi)\right)^2\end{array}} \tag{3.2}$$

In Fig. 3.3b, $\theta$ represents the angle made by link BC with the horizontal. Link BC may be rotated by varying the length of the linear actuator. Also, $\psi$ is angle between link CD with the vertical when $\theta = 0°$. $\psi$ may be varied as per the user comfort. The length of the linear actuator ($L_a$) is given by Eq. 3.2.

### 3.3.2 Linear Actuator Stroke Length

The inclination angle of the proposed system can be adjusted by changing the length of the linear actuator connected to the rear wheel. This section focuses on deriving the operating range of the actuator. The maximum elongation limit of the linear actuator is derived from the situation when the wheelchair climbs on obstacles, whereas the minimum length is derived from the condition of climbing down the obstacle.

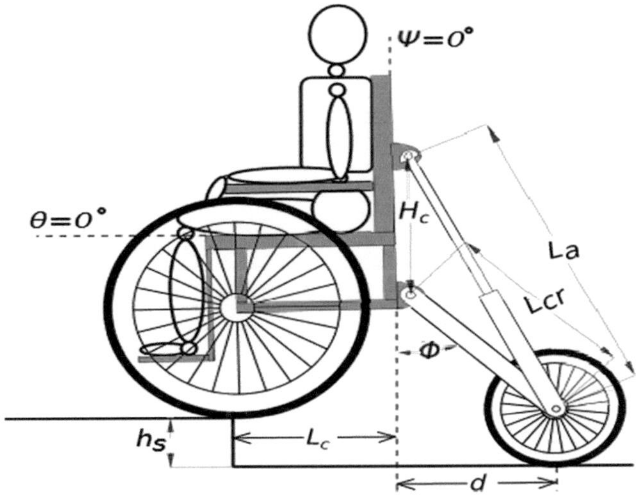


**Fig. 3.4** Schematic for actuator length calculation while ascending

#### 3.3.2.1 Case 1: Ascent of the Wheelchair

As shown in Fig. 3.4, the maximum required length of the linear actuator for successfully climbing an obstacle while maintaining the inclination angle depends on the obstacle's height. The equation for the maximum required length of the linear actuator is given by Eq. 3.3.

$\phi$ Minimum angle between crank with vertical

It may be noticed that the wheelchair will be more stable for a higher value of $\phi$. Moreover, the value of $\phi$ should never become negative. However, increasing $\phi$ will result in an increase in the length of the crank and the linear actuator.

$$
\begin{aligned}
L_{\mathrm{cr}} &= \frac{h_s + R + L_c \sin\theta - r}{\cos\phi} \\
d &= \sqrt{L_{\mathrm{cr}}^2 + (R + L_c \sin\theta - r)^2} \\
L_a &= \sqrt{\begin{array}{c}(d - H_c \sin(\theta + \psi))^2 + \\ (h_s + R + L_c \sin\theta + H_c \cos(\theta + \psi) - r)^2\end{array}}
\end{aligned} \tag{3.3}
$$

#### 3.3.2.2 Case 2: Descent of the Wheelchair

Likewise, the minimum allowable length of the actuator link is determined from the descending scenario, where the front wheel has completed the descent, and the rear wheel remains on the elevated plane. Equation of finding actuator length in this condition is represented by Eq. 3.4. Figure 3.5 presents a schematic representation for determining the minimum length of the actuator link.

$$
\begin{aligned}
L_{\mathrm{cr}} &= \frac{R + L_c \sin\theta - h_s - r}{\cos\phi} \\
d &= \sqrt{L_{\mathrm{cr}}^2 - (R + L_c \sin\theta - h_s - r)^2} \\
L_a &= \sqrt{\begin{array}{c}(d - H_c \sin(\theta + \psi))^2 + \\ (R + L_c \sin\theta - h_s + H_c \cos(\theta + \psi) - r)^2\end{array}}
\end{aligned} \tag{3.4}
$$

Calculating the maximum and minimum length of $L_a$ is an important design parameter for the safe operation of the wheelchair on obstacles.

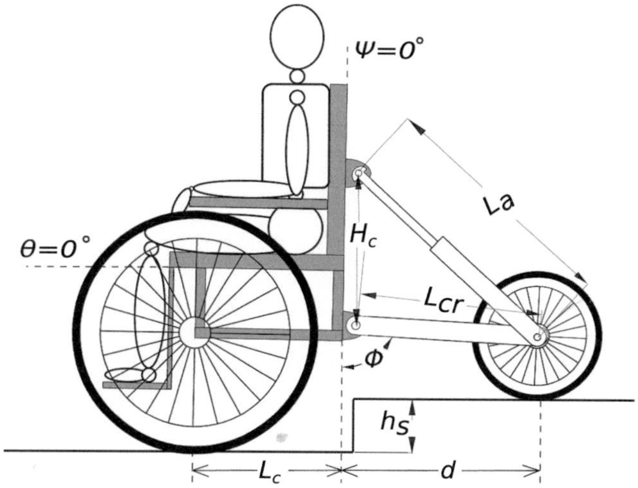


**Fig. 3.5** Schematic for actuator length calculation while descending

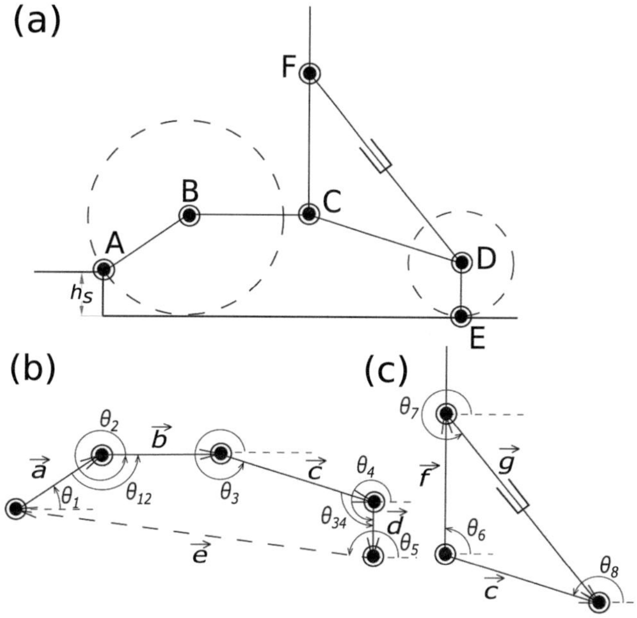


**Fig. 3.6** Kinematic model of the wheelchair; **a** schematic of the wheelchair; **b** kinematic model of chain 1; **c** kinematic model of chain 2

### 3.3.3 Kinematics of the System

Kinematic analysis is performed to establish the relationship of the relative motion between the system's links. The simplified kinematic model of the proposed system is represented using rigid links, as shown in Fig. 3.6a. In this model, the front wheels are represented by link AB and the rear wheels are link DE. Assuming that the wheel rolls without slipping on the obstacle edge, the contact point of the step's edge and the wheel is considered a hinge joint for analytical purposes.

As the wheels move along a horizontal surface, the links connecting the wheel centre to the contact point are assumed to remain perpendicular to the ground. To simplify calculations, the system is divided into two kinematic chains, as illustrated in Fig. 3.6b and c. Equations illustrating the position, velocity, and acceleration of the links are provided in the following subsection.

#### 3.3.3.1 Position, Velocity, and Acceleration

Equations 3.6–3.8 illustrate the position, velocity and acceleration of the links. Each equation consists of a pair of equation, representing the two kinematic chains.

Figure 3.6b illustrates chain 1 and Fig. 3.6c shows chain 2. Length of links AB, BC, CD, DE and DF are system parameters. The location of point A and F are given by $(x_a, y_a)$ and $(x_e, y_e)$.

$$
\begin{aligned}
|\vec{e}| &= \sqrt{(x_a - x_e)^2 + (y_a - y_e)^2} \\
\theta_5 &= \arctan\left(\frac{y_a - y_e}{x_a - x_e}\right) \\
\theta_{12} &= \theta_2 - (\pi + \theta_1) \\
\theta_{34} &= \theta_4 - \theta_3 + \pi
\end{aligned} \tag{3.5}
$$

$\theta_{12}$ and $\theta_{34}$ are the input angles. The relationship between input angles and $\theta_2$, $\theta_3$ are given by Eq. 3.5. $\theta_2$ and $\theta_3$ are obtained by equating the real and imaginary parts of the position equation for chain 1.

Likewise, by comparing the real and imaginary components of the position equation for chain 2, the magnitude of $\vec{g}$ and $\theta_7$ is determined. The position equations are provided by:

$$
\begin{aligned}
&\vec{a}e^{j\theta_1} + \vec{b}e^{j\theta_2} + \vec{c}e^{j\theta_3} + \vec{d}e^{j\theta_4} + \vec{e}e^{j\theta_5} = 0 \\
&-\vec{c}e^{j\theta_8} + \vec{f}e^{j\theta_6} + \vec{g}e^{j\theta_7} = 0
\end{aligned} \tag{3.6}
$$

The velocity equations may be written as:

$$
\begin{aligned}
&\vec{a}j\omega_1 e^{j\theta_1} + \vec{b}j\omega_2 e^{j\theta_2} + \vec{c}j\omega_3 e^{j\theta_3} + \vec{d}j\omega_4 e^{j\theta_4} + \left(\vec{e}j\omega_5 - \dot{\vec{e}}\right)e^{j\theta_5} = 0 \\
&-\vec{c}j\omega_8 e^{j\theta_8} + \vec{f}j\omega_6 e^{j\theta_6} + \left(\vec{g}j\omega_7 - \dot{\vec{g}}\right)e^{j\theta_7} = 0
\end{aligned} \tag{3.7}
$$

The acceleration equation may be written as:

$$
\begin{aligned}
&\vec{a}\left(j\alpha_1 - \omega_1^2\right)e^{j\theta_1} + \vec{b}\left(j\alpha_2 - \omega_2^2\right)e^{j\theta_2} + \vec{c}\left(j\alpha_3 - \omega_3^2\right)e^{j\theta_3} + \vec{d}\left(j\alpha_4 - \omega_4^2\right)e^{j\theta_4} \\
&\quad + \left(\vec{e}\left(j\alpha_5 - \omega_5^2\right) + 2\dot{\vec{e}}j\omega_5 - \ddot{\vec{e}}\right)e^{j\theta_5} = 0 \\
&-\vec{c}\left(j\alpha_8 - \omega_8^2\right)e^{j\theta_8} + \vec{f}\left(j\alpha_6 - \omega_6^2\right)e^{j\theta_6} + \left(\vec{g}\left(j\alpha_7 - \omega_7^2\right) + 2\dot{\vec{g}}\omega_7 - \ddot{\vec{g}}\right)e^{j\theta_7} = 0
\end{aligned} \tag{3.8}
$$

Solving the velocity and acceleration equations, the unknown $\omega_2, \omega_3, \omega_7, \alpha_2, \alpha_3, \alpha_7$ and magnitude of $\dot{\vec{g}}$ and $\ddot{\vec{g}}$ are determined. These angular velocities and accelerations are utilized in the dynamic analysis to determine the joint forces.

### 3.3.4 System Dynamics Analysis

This section explores the dynamic equations that govern the system proposed in this study. These equations are essential for evaluating the forces acting on various links due to the combined weight of the rider and the system, as well as the system's movement over obstacles. The derivation of these equations is based on the Newton–Euler method, which provides a systematic approach for analysing the system's dynamics.

#### 3.3.4.1 Equation of Motion of the Wheelchair

The system dynamic model was developed by taking into account a scenario where the front wheels are the verge of rolling over the edges of obstacles. Various phases of the wheelchair's motion may be represented by considering the angles, $\theta_1$ and $\theta_4$ to 90° or 270°, respectively. For instance, when the front wheel is moving on horizontal plane, $\theta_1$ is considered as 90°. Similarly, depending on whether the wheel on plane motion or climbing motion, setting the value of $\theta_1$ and $\theta_4$, respective equation of motion of the system may be derived.

Figure 3.7 represents the free-body diagram of each link of the system. All link numbers are encircled. Forces on each node are represented by 'F'. 'a' represents the linear accelerations of links. '$T_{12}$' and '$T_{34}$' shows the torque applied between link 1 and 2 and link 3 and 4, respectively. 'I' and '$\alpha$', represent the mass moment of inertia and angular acceleration of the links. The mass of human and link 2 are combined and considered to be acting at point 'G'. The planar equilibrium equations for different members of the system are given through Eqs. 3.9–3.15.

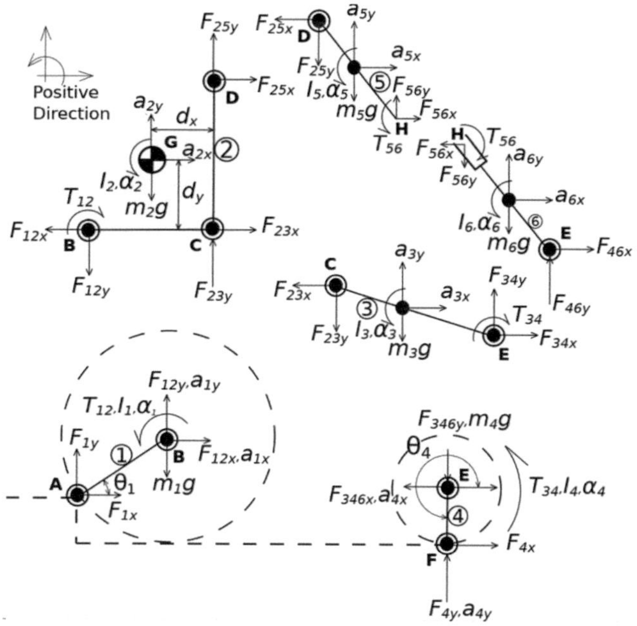


**Fig. 3.7** Free body diagram of different members of the proposed wheelchair

Link 1

$$
\begin{aligned}
&F_{1x} + F_{12x} = m_1 a_{1x} \\
&F_{1y} + F_{12y} = m_1\left(a_{1y} + g\right) \\
&F_{1x} d_{\mathrm{AB},y} - F_{1y} d_{\mathrm{AB},x} + T_{12} = I_1 \alpha_1
\end{aligned} \tag{3.9}
$$

Link 2

$$
\begin{aligned}
&- F_{12x} + F_{23x} + F_{25x} = m_2 a_{2x} - F_{12y} + F_{23y} + F_{25y} = m_2\left(a_{2y} + g\right) \\
&- F_{12x} d_{\mathrm{BG},y} + F_{12y} d_{\mathrm{BG},x} + F_{23x} d_{\mathrm{CG},y} + F_{23y} d_{\mathrm{CG},x} \\
&\quad - F_{25x} d_{\mathrm{DG},y} + F_{25y} d_{\mathrm{DG},x} - T_{12} = I_2 \alpha_2
\end{aligned} \tag{3.10}
$$

Link 3

$$
\begin{aligned}
&- F_{23x} + F_{34x} = m_3 a_{3x} \\
&- F_{23y} + F_{34y} = m_3\left(a_{3y} + g\right)
\end{aligned} \tag{3.11}
$$

Link 4

$$
\begin{aligned}
&- F_{346x} + F_{4x} = m_4 a_{3x} \\
&- F_{346y} + F_{4y} = m_4\left(a_{4y} + g\right) \\
&F_{4x} d_{\mathrm{EF},y} = I_4 \alpha_4 - T_{34}
\end{aligned} \tag{3.12}
$$

Link 5

$$
\begin{aligned}
&- F_{25x} + F_{56x} = m_5 a_{5x} \\
&- F_{25y} + F_{56y} = m_5\left(a_{5y} + g\right) \\
&F_{25x} \frac{d_{\mathrm{DH},y}}{2} + F_{25y} \frac{d_{\mathrm{DH},x}}{2} + F_{56x} \frac{d_{\mathrm{DH},y}}{2} + F_{56x} \frac{d_{\mathrm{DH},x}}{2} - T_{56} = I_5 \alpha_5
\end{aligned} \tag{3.13}
$$

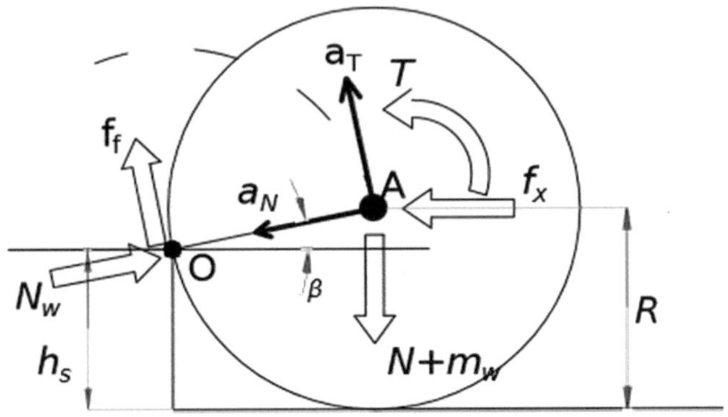


**Fig. 3.8** Free body diagram of wheel when wheel rolls over an obstacle. *Note* The contact force between the wheel and the horizontal plane is ignored as the wheel will be momentarily out of contact during roll over

Link 6

$$
\begin{aligned}
&- F_{56x} + F_{46x} = m_6 a_{6x} \\
&- F_{56y} + F_{46y} = m_6 \big(a_{6y} + g\big) \\
&F_{56x}\frac{d_{\mathrm{EH},y}}{2} + F_{56y}\frac{d_{\mathrm{EH},x}}{2} + F_{46x}\frac{d_{\mathrm{EH},y}}{2} + F_{46x}\frac{d_{\mathrm{EH},x}}{2} + T_{56} = I_6\alpha_6
\end{aligned} \tag{3.14}
$$

Additional equations

$$
\begin{aligned}
&F_{34} + F_{46x} - F_{346x} = 0 \\
&F_{34y} + F_{46y} - F_{346y} = 0
\end{aligned} \tag{3.15}
$$

#### 3.3.4.2 Equation of Motion of Wheel

This section focuses on deriving the wheel's equation of motion. Figure 3.8 illustrates the free-body diagram (FBD) of a wheel subjected to a torque (T) at its centre. The wheel has a radius (R) and a mass ($m_W$) and is attempting to overcome an obstacle of height ($h_s$). The external forces acting at the wheel's centre include $f_x$ and N, which result in a normal reaction force ($N_W$). The wheel's motion due to the applied torque produces radial ($a_N$) and tangential ($a_T$) accelerations.

The angle $\beta$represents the inclination between the horizontal surface and the line connecting the instantaneous centre of rolling to the centre of the wheel. If the wheel moves forward without slipping at the contact point (O), then the relative velocity at this point is zero. As a result, static friction ($f_f$) is the only force responsible for the forward movement of the wheel, acting in the direction of motion. The equations of motion governing the wheel's behaviour are provided in Eqs. 3.16–3.18.

$$
\begin{aligned}
&N_w \cos\beta - f_f \sin\beta - m_w a_T \sin\beta - m_w a_N \cos\beta - f_x = 0 \\
&N_w \sin\beta + f_f \cos\beta - m_w a_T \cos\beta - m_w a_N \sin\beta - m_w - N = 0 \\
&T - f_f \times \mathrm{OA} = I_w \alpha
\end{aligned} \tag{3.16}
$$

## 3.4 Prototype Development

To demonstrate the working of the proposed system, a full-scale prototype is developed. The development of the prototype of the proposed system is subdivided into two groups. In first part mechanical parts, design and fabrication are discussed whereas, in the second part, electronics involved in the prototype are discussed. In the following subsections, the two parts are discussed in detail.

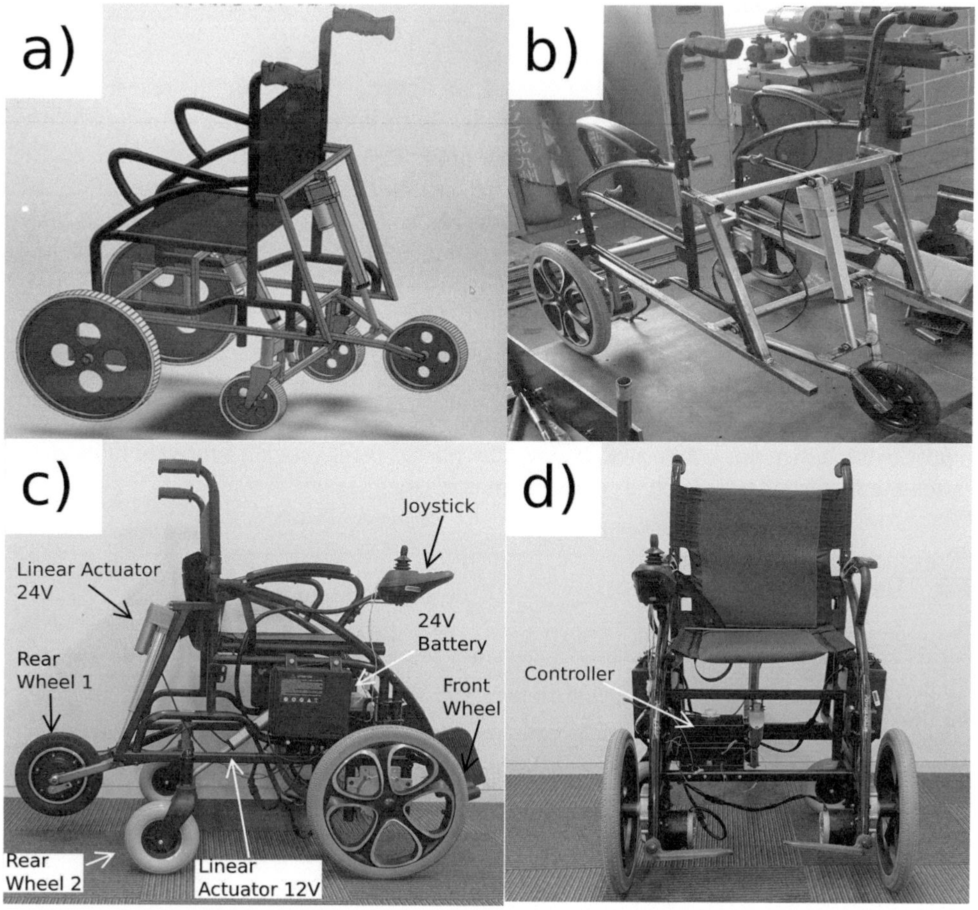


**Fig. 3.9** Prototype design and development of the wheelchair; **a** 3-D model; **b** partial fabrication; **c** parts and components description (side view); **d** front view

### 3.4.1 Mechanical Design and Fabrication

For the development of the full-scale prototype of the proposed system, a 3-D design of the system is developed using SOLIDWORKS. Figure 3.9a shows the designed 3-D model of the wheelchair. Figure 3.9b illustrates an image of the wheelchair when the development process is partially completed. Figure 3.9c and d represent the side view and front view of the fully developed wheelchair, respectively. It may be noticed from Fig. 3.9c that the wheelchair is equipped with two types of rear wheels, rear-wheel 1 and rear wheel 2. Rear-wheel 1 is operated by a powerful linear actuator, i.e., 24 V linear actuator, whereas rear wheel 2 is connected to a 12 V linear actuator. Since the rear wheel 1 assembly plays a key role in regulating the change in the wheelchair's inclination angle, a 24 Volts powerful actuator is used. While the wheelchair is moving on the plane surface, the rear end of the wheelchair is supported by rear wheel 2 assembly, and the rear wheel 1 assembly is kept in the retracted position. Rear-wheel 2 are a set of caster wheels that are used while turning left or right. Rear-wheel 1 is engaged only at the time of overcoming an obstacle. At that moment rear wheel 2 will be retracted using a 12 V linear actuator, as it may hinder the ascending or descending motion. Description of major parts of the developed wheelchair is shown in Table 3.1. In the next section, we will discuss the design and development of the controller for the proposed obstacle-avoiding wheelchair.

### 3.4.2 Electronics of the Prototype

In Fig. 3.10 various components used to develop the controller are shown. The entire controller is subdivided into two parts, that is, the power system, and actuator control system. The wheelchair is powered by two 24 V batteries which are connected in parallel. Two linear actuators of 24–12 V are powered by two DC-DC buck converters, which are connected in series (as shown in Fig. 3.10). The first converter outputs stable 24 V, which is used to power the 24 V linear actuator and as the input to the second buck converter. The output stable 12 V from second buck converter is used to power the 12 V linear actuator.

Moreover, the front brushed direct current (DC) motors and rear brushless direct current (BLDC) hub motors are powered by the stable 24 V output from the first buck converter.

Remaining components are used to control the linear actuators and the rear hub motor. The main micro-controller used in the system is an Arduino Uno R3. The joystick is used to drive the front motors of the wheelchair. The three-way switch is used to toggle between ascending, descending, and plane mode of the wheelchair. Usually, the toggle switch will be in plane mode, however, to overcome obstacles the user will need to switch to ascending/descending mode (depending upon the climbing conditions). The 12 V linear actuator is controlled by the L289N motor controller. Similarly, the 24 V linear actuator is controlled by a 24 V motor controller. To control the direction of the 24 V linear actuator two MOSFET transistors (IRF520) are used. The position sensor of the linear actuator helps to precisely detect the length of the actuator. An IMU (MPU6050) is utilized to detect changes in the wheelchair's inclination angle. This sensor is comprised of three gyroscopes and three accelerometers. Inputs from these six sensors are used to detect any change in the inclination angle of the wheelchair. In the prototype, a hall sensor-based BLDC hub motor is used, which is powered by 24 V input and controlled by Arduino Uno. Before climbing over an obstacle, once the rider selects the ascending mode and the rear hub motor is engaged, the power supply to the hub motor is activated. As the rider pushes the joystick for forward motion, the signal from the joystick is sensed by the microcontroller and actuates the hub motor.

## 3.5 Results and Discussion

In this section the results of simulations and experiments are explained. Using the model illustrated in Sect. 3.3, simulations are performed to analyse the behaviour of the proposed wheelchair. In the following subsection the results of the simulations are illustrated in detail.

### 3.5.1 Simulation Results

Simulations are performed to analyse the system while climbing over an obstacle. Table 3.2 shows the dimension of the links considered for the simulation. The mass of the rider is considered as 100 kg and the co-efficient of static friction is considered as 0.6.

Figure 3.11 illustrates the various forces on the front and rear wheels. The inclination angle of the wheelchair is varied from 0° to 10° and the variation in forces is plotted. It may be noticed that as the inclination increases, the load shared by the front wheel centre decreases. Since the entire load is shared between front and rear wheel centres, as the load at the front-wheel decreases, the load at the rear-wheel increases. Since the load at the front wheel is reduced by inclining the wheelchair, this accounts for the low torque required by the front wheel to climb up the obstacle. Moreover, as the load at the rear wheel increases, the horizontal push (which is directly proportional to the normal load) by the rear wheel also increases. This collectively reduces the torque needed at the front wheels to roll over the obstacle, as illustrated in Fig. 3.12.

**Table 3.1** Description of parts of the prototype of the wheelchair

| Parts name | Description |
|---|---|
| Front wheels | Radius-200 mm |
| Caster wheels | Radius-90 mm |
| Controller | Arduino Uno ($\mu C$) |
| Power supply | Two 24 V batteries |
| Front motor | 24VDC, 250W, 1800 RPM(Max.),16.5:1 (Gear Ratio) |
| Hub motor | 24 V BLDC, 350W, 800 RPM(Max.) |
| IMU | MPU6050 |
| Linear actuator 1 | 200 mm (Stroke) 2000 N (Max. Load) |
| Linear actuator 2 | 12 V, 150 mm (Stroke) 500 N (Max. Load) |

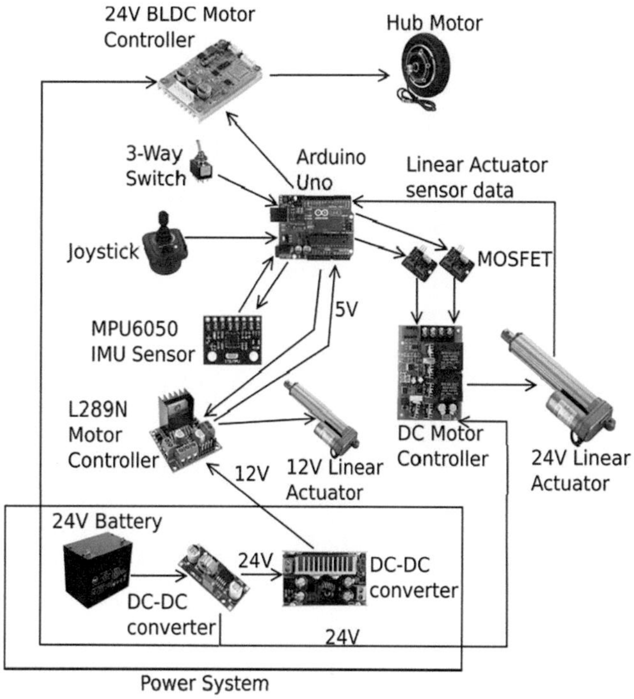


**Fig. 3.10** Various electronic components used to develop the control system of the wheelchair

**Table 3.2** Dimension of members of wheelchair used for the simulation (Refer Fig. 3.7)

| Link | Dimensions (mm) | Link | Dimensions (mm) |
|---|---|---|---|
| AB | 200 | EF | 100 |
| BC | 400 | CD | 600 |
| CE | 600 | $h_s$ | 35 |
| $d_x$ | 100 | $d_y$ | 300 |

### 3.5.2 Experiment Results

In this section, the results of the experiments on the developed wheelchair are discussed. Figure 3.13 shows the snapshots of the experiments while the wheelchair is climbing on an obstacle. In the experiment, a block of 35 mm height is considered as the obstacle. The schematic illustrating the ascending process is illustrated in Fig. 3.14. In Fig. 3.13a shows, the location of the rear caster wheel, hub motor (attached to front frame with slider-crank mechanism), and the obstacle block. Figure 3.13b shows that before climbing up the obstacle, the rider switches to the climbing mode. The climbing mode consists of three

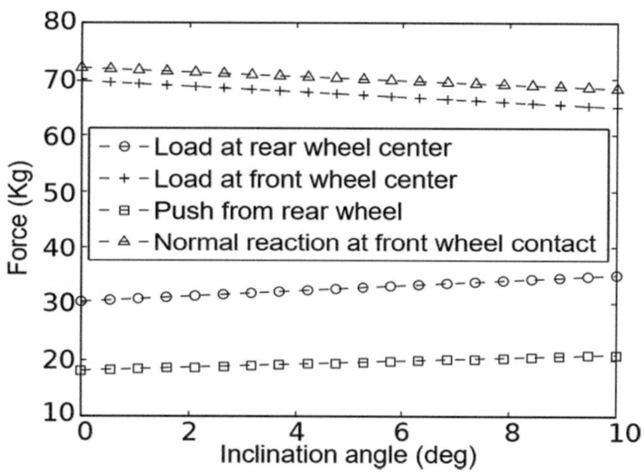


**Fig. 3.11** Forces at front and rear wheels with respect to variation in inclination angle

steps. First, the rear hub motor is engaged as shown in Fig. 3.13b, then the caster wheels are disengaged, which is shown in Fig. 3.13c. Finally, by actuating the linear actuator the wheelchair inclination angle is maintained horizontal to the ground. Figure 3.13e and f show successful climbing of the wheelchair over the obstacle as the rider actuates the front motors with the help of a joystick. The rear hub motor provides an additional forward force to aid the front motors to overcome the obstacle.

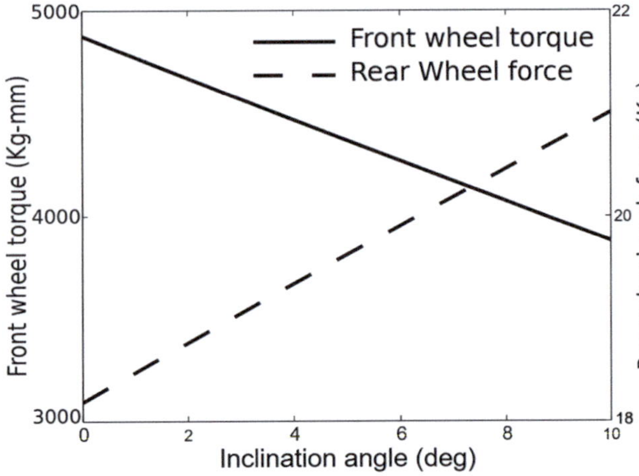


**Fig. 3.12** Variation of required torque at front wheel and pushing force from rear wheel with respect to the change in inclination angle

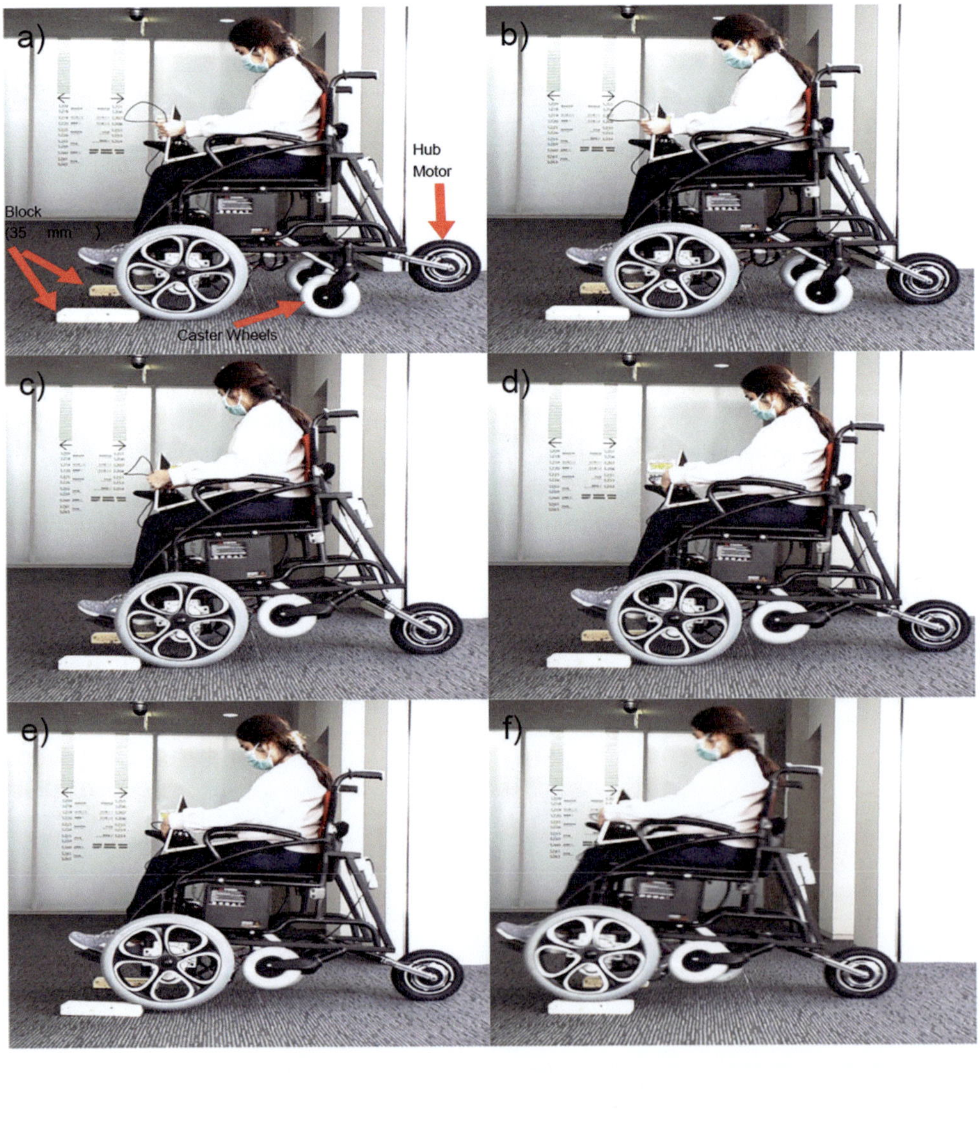


**Fig. 3.13** Few frames of the experiment of wheelchair during climbing on an obstacle

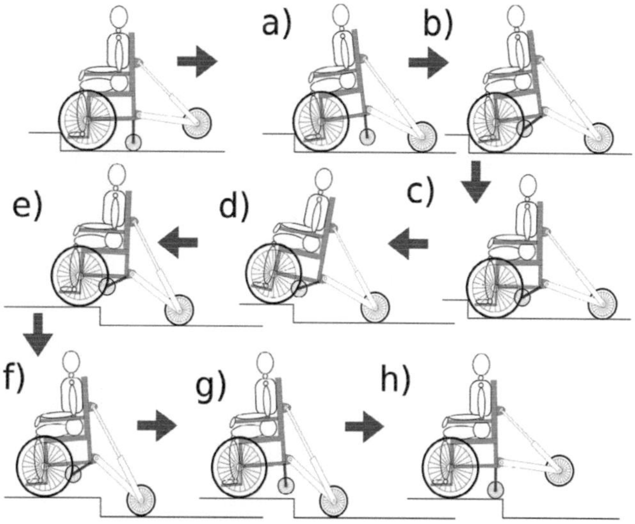


**Fig. 3.14** Schematic illustrating the ascending of the proposed wheelchair

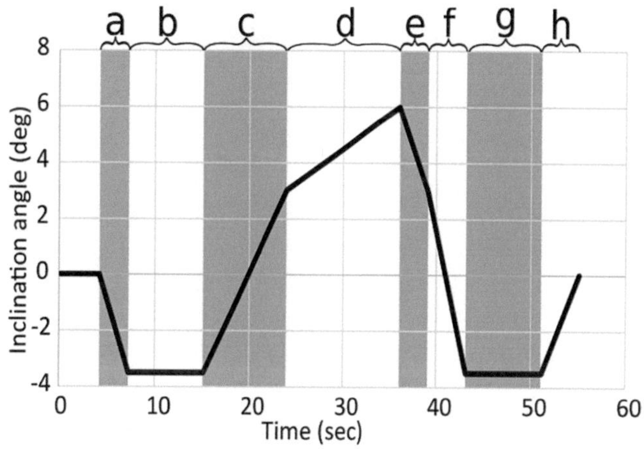


**Fig. 3.15** Variation of inclination angle during ascending with control

Figure 3.15 shows the variation of the inclination angle of the wheelchair during the entire climbing process. The entire process is divided into eight zones. During zone 'a', the hub motor is lowered so that the caster wheels can be retracted, which is represented by zone 'b'. Zone 'c' illustrates the auto-correction of the wheelchair angle to a preset angle (preset is set to 3°). Then the ascending phase of the wheelchair is shown by zone 'd' in which the inclination angle of the wheelchair raises to 6°. Immediately after that, the auto-correction system rearranged itself to the set angle of 3°, which is shown by the zone 'e'. Once the front wheel climbs over the obstacle the plain mode of the wheelchair is activated in which the caster wheels are deployed, and the hub wheel is retracted. This is shown by the zone's 'f', 'g', and 'h'.

Figure 3.16 shows a few of the snapshots taken during climbing down on an obstacle. In this experiment, the obstacle height is 70 mm. It may be noticed from Fig. 3.16a–d, that during the descent the caster wheels are engaged. In Fig. 3.16b illustrates the scenario when the front wheels are about to roll down from the edge of the obstacle and the descent has started. Figure 3.16c shows that the front wheel has completed the descent whereas the rear wheels are still on the elevated side of the obstacle. Because of the elevation difference of the rear and front wheel, it may be noticed that the inclination angle of the wheelchair reduces to −6° (negative). This inclination angle is directly influenced by the height of the obstacle. More the height lower will be the inclination angle. Finally Fig. 3.16d shows when entire wheelchair have completed the descent.

Figure 3.17 shows the snapshots taken during the experiment when the wheelchair is descending over an obstacle and the inclination angle of the wheelchair is controlled by actuating a linear actuator that connects the rear wheel to the front frame of the wheelchair. The schematic illustrating the ascending process is illustrated in Fig. 3.18. From Fig. 3.17a–j, the entire process of descent operation is shown. Figure 3.17a shows that as the rider reaches towards the edge of the obstacle, the rider switches the mode of the wheelchair to descent mode. Like the ascent mode, the descent mode comprises three steps. As shown in Fig. 3.17b, the first step engages the rear hub wheel which is attached to the front frame by a slider-crank

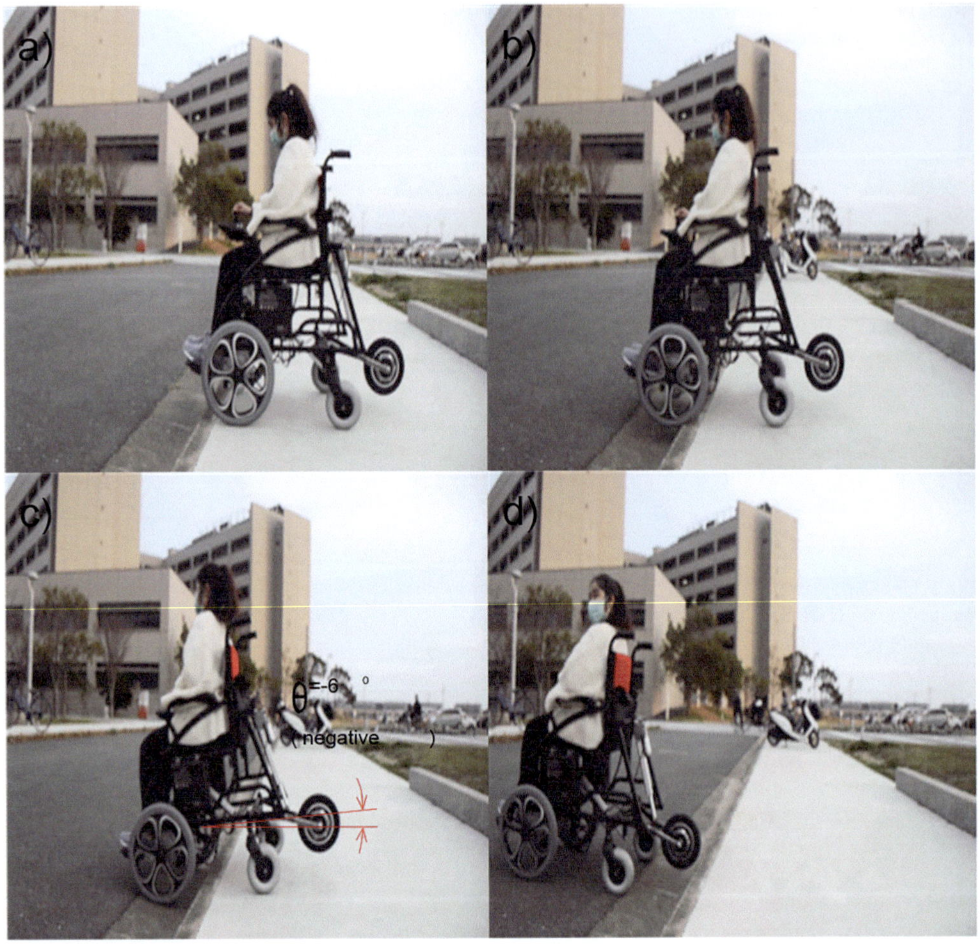


**Fig. 3.16** Few frames of the experiment of wheelchair during descending on an obstacle without control

mechanism. In Fig. 3.17c, it may be noticed that the caster wheels are disengaged. Figure 3.17d shows that the length of the linear actuator is adjusted, which in turns varies the inclination angle of the wheelchair to maintain desired angle. Figure 3.17e indicates that the front wheels are at the edge of the obstacle and the descent of the wheelchair has started. In Fig. 3.17f, it may be observed that the front wheels have completed the descent process whereas the rear wheel is still on the elevated side of the obstacle. It may be noticed that, as compared to descent without controlling the inclination angle, during controlled operation, the inclination angle of the wheelchair is 1° (which is safer as compared to uncontrolled operation). Figure 3.17g shows that entire wheelchair have overcome the obstacle and the rider switches to plane mode, in which caster wheels will be engaged and the rear wheel with hub motor will be disengaged. The processes of returning to plane mode are shown through Fig. 3.17h–j.

The variation in inclination angle during descending of an obstacle in both with and without the proposed mechanism is shown in Fig. 3.19. As shown in the figure, the entire process is divided into 10 zones. Similar to ascending case, zone 'a', 'b' and 'c' illustrate the process where the hub wheel is engaged, and the caster wheels are retracted. In zone 'd', the front wheel of the wheelchair descends the obstacle. It may be noticed that the inclination angle change to −6° when the proposed mechanism is not used, whereas when the mechanism is used the inclination angle of the wheelchair is 1° after landing of the front wheel of the wheelchair. Immediately after that, the wheelchair inclination angle is auto corrected to 3°, which is shown through Zone 'e'. Zone 'f' illustrates the descend of the rear wheel. In zone 'g' the auto-correction of inclination angle is shown. Zone 'h', 'i', and 'j' illustrate the re-engagement of caster wheels and the retraction of the hub wheel.

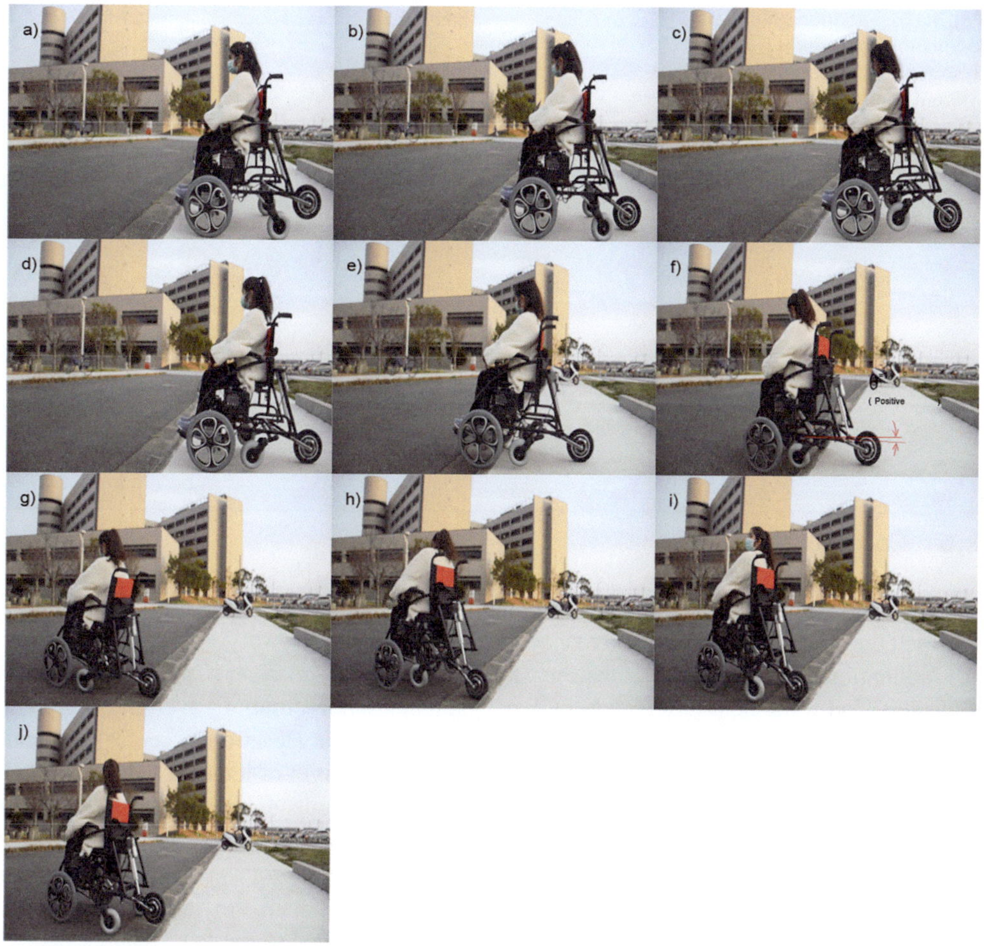


**Fig. 3.17** Few frames of the experiment of wheelchair during descending on an obstacle with control

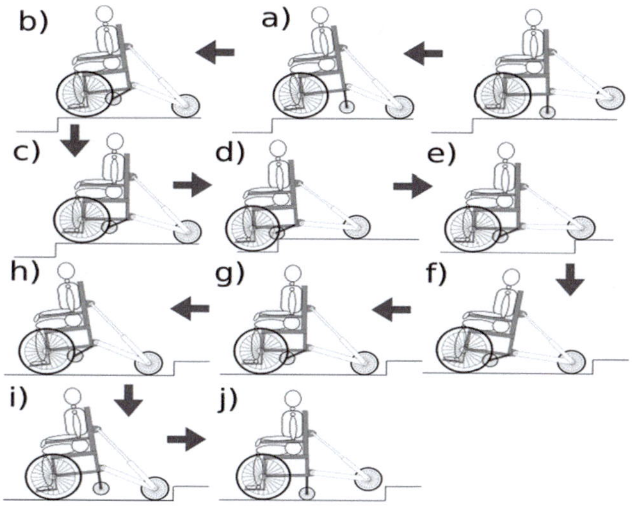


**Fig. 3.18** Schematic illustrating the descending of the proposed wheelchair

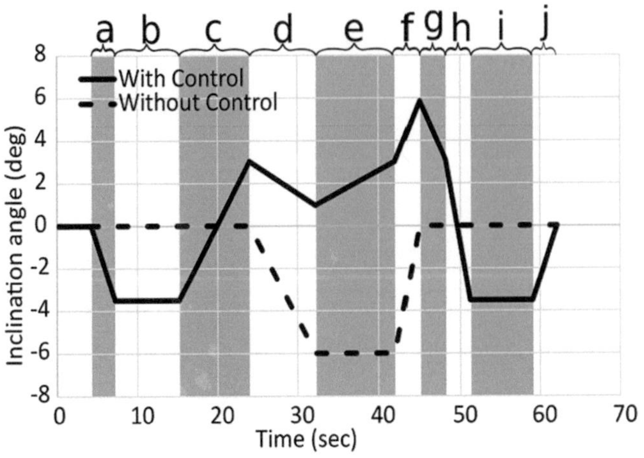


**Fig. 3.19** Variation of inclination angle during descending with control and without control

## 3.6 Conclusion

In this article, a minimalistic obstacle overcoming wheelchair is proposed. A mechanism is proposed so that the centre distance between the centres of the front and rear wheels can be altered. By varying the centre distance between front and rear wheels, the inclination angle of the wheelchair is varied. In the proposed system, the rear wheel is attached to the front frame of the wheelchair with the help of a slider-crank mechanism. While climbing over an obstacle with a system in which front and rear wheels are attached by rigid links, due to the difference in elevation of centre of front and rear wheels, the wheelchair's inclination angle changes significantly. By controlling the length of linear actuator in the proposed wheelchair, the variation in inclination angle of the wheelchair is minimized. Experiments are carried out to demonstrate the proposed system. It was found that the proposed wheelchair successfully climbed up an obstacle of 35 mm height. Moreover, while descending from an elevation of 70 mm, the variation in inclination angle of the proposed wheelchair was limited to $1^\circ$ as compared to $-6^\circ$ while descending with rigid wheelchair. In the proposed mechanism, the rider must select the modes depending on ascending, descending, or plane motion. In future, sensors will be attached to the wheelchair to detect the obstacle and autonomously changes the mode of the wheelchair depending on the ascending or descending situations. Also, the design will be further improved so that the wheelchair can climb up or down the stairs.

**Acknowledgements** The authors are highly thankful for the subjects involved in this study for their cooperation.

## References

1. Anderson GF, Hussey PS (2000) Population aging: a comparison among industrialized countries. Health affairs (Project Hope) 19(3):191–203
2. Okuno E (1998) Disability statistics in Japan
3. Batavia M (1998) The wheelchair evaluation: a practical guide. Butterworth-Heinemann Medical
4. Lawn MJ, Sakai T, Kuroiwa M, Ishimatsu T (2001) Development and practical application of a stairclimbing wheelchair in Nagasaki. Int J Human-Friendly Welfare Robot Syst, pp 33–39
5. Hirose S, Fukushima EF, Damoto R, Nakamoto H (2001) Design of terrain adaptive versatile crawler vehicle HELIOS-VI. IEEE Int Conf Intell Robot Syst 3:1540–1545
6. Yu S, Wang T, Li X, Yao C, Wang Z, Zhi D (2010) Configuration and tip-over stability analysis for stair-climbing of a new-style wheelchair robot. In: IEEE International Conference on Mechatronics and Automation (ICMA), pp 1387–1392
7. Sugahara Y, Ohta A, Hashimoto K, Sunazuka H, Kawase M, Tanaka C, Lim H-O, Takanishi A (2005) Walking up and down stairs carrying a human by a biped locomotor with parallel mechanism. In: IEEE/RSJ International Conference on Intelligent Robots and Systems, pp 1489–1494
8. Yuan J, Hirose S (2004) Research on leg-wheel hybrid stair-climbing robot, ZeroCarrier. IEEE International Conference on Robotics and Biomimetics, pp 654–659
9. Bang Y-B, Lee C-H, Yoo J-H, Lee K-M, Kim I-S (2011) Two legged stair-climbing wheelchair and its stair dimension measurement using distance sensors. In: 11th International conference on control, automation and systems, pp 1788–1791
10. Wang H, He L, Li Q, Zhang W, Zhang D, Xu P (2014) Research on a kind of leg-wheel stair-climbing wheelchair, In: IEEE international conference on mechatronics and automation, pp 2101–2105
11. Misawa R (1986) Stair-climbing wheelchair carrier

12. Lawn MJ, Ishimatsu T (2003) Modeling of a stair-climbing wheelchair mechanism with high single-step capability. IEEE Trans Neural Syst Rehabil Eng 11:3(323–332)
13. Liu J, Wu Y, Guo J, Chen Q (2015) High-order sliding mode-based synchronous control of a novel stair-climbing wheelchair robot. J Control Sci Eng, pp 1–16
14. Morales R, Feliu V, Gonzalez A, Pintado P (2006) Kinematic model of a new staircase climbing wheelchair and its experimental validation. Int J Robot Res 25(9):825–841
15. Morales R, Feliu V, Gonzalez A, Pintado P (2006) Coordinated motion of a new staircase climbing wheelchair with increased passenger comfort. In: Proceedings—IEEE international conference on robotics and automation, pp 3995–4001
16. Morales R, Gonzalez A, Feliu V, Pintado P (2007) Environment adaptation of a new staircase climbing wheelchair. Auton Robot 23(4):275–292
17. Gonzalez A, Ottaviano E, Ceccarelli M (2009) On the kinematic functionality of a fourbar based mechanism for guiding wheels in climbing steps and obstacles. Mech Mach Theory 44(8):1507–1523
18. Morales R, Feliu V, Gonzalez A (2010) Optimized obstacle avoidance trajectory generation for a reconfigurable staircase climbing wheelchair. Robot Auton Syst 58(1):97–114
19. Chocoteco J, Morales R, Feliu V, Sanchez L (2016) Trajectory planning for a stair-climbing mobility system using laser distance sensors. IEEE Syst J 10(3):944956
20. Baishya NJ, Bhattacharya B, Ogai H, Tatsumi K (2021) Design of an anti-slip mechanism for wheels of step climbing robots. Actuators 10(10):259. https://doi.org/10.3390/act10100259
21. Shino M, Tomokuni N, Murata G, Segawa M (2014) Wheeled inverted pendulum type robotic wheelchair with integrated control of seat slider and rotary link between wheels for climbing stairs. In: IEEE international workshop on advanced robotics and its social impacts, pp 121–126
22. Ghani NMA, Nasir ANK, Tokhi MO (2014) Optimization of fuzzy logic scaling parameters with spiral dynamic algorithm in controlling a stair climbing wheelchair: ascending task. In: 19th international conference on methods and models in automation and robotics (MMAR), pp 776–781
23. Chen CT, Pham HV (2009) Design and fabrication of a statically stable stairclimbing robotic wheelchair. Ind Robot 36(6):562–569
24. Sugahara Y, Yonezawa N, Kosuge N (2010) A novel stair-climbing wheelchair with transformable wheeled four-bar linkages. In: IEEE/RSJ 2010 international conference on intelligent robots and systems (IROS), pp 3333–3339
25. Quaglia G, Maffiodo D, Franco W, Appendino S, Oderio R (2009) The Epi.q-1 hybrid mobile robot. Int J Robot Res 29(1):81–91
26. Quaglia G, Franco W, Oderio R (2009) Wheelchair.q, a mechanical concept for a stair climbing wheelchair. In: IEEE international conference on robotics and biomimetics (ROBIO), pp 800–805
27. Quaglia G, Franco W, Oderio R (2011) Wheelchair.q, a motorized wheelchair with stair climbing ability. Mech Mach Theory 46(11):1601–1609
28. Quaglia G, Oderio R, Bruzzone L, Razzoli R (2013) A modular approach for a family of ground mobile robots. Int J Adv Robot Syst 10
29. Quaglia G, Nisi M (2014) Design of a reconfiguration mechanism for an electric stair-climbing wheelchair. In: Proceedings of the ASME 2014 international mechanical engineering congress and exposition, pp 1–10
30. Quaglia G, Matteo N (2015) Design and construction of a new version of the EPI.Q UGV for monitoring and surveillance tasks. In: Proceedings of the ASME 2015 international mechanical engineering congress and exposition, pp 1–8
31. Quaglia G, Franco W, Nisi M (2015) Evolution of Wheelchair.q, a stair-climbing wheelchair. In: The 14th IFToMM world congress
32. Quaglia G, Nisi M (2017) Design of a self-leveling cam mechanism for a stair climbing wheelchair. Mech Mach Theory 112:84–104
33. Wada M (2008) A 4WD omnidirectional wheelchair with enhanced step climbing capability. J Robot Mechatron 20(6):846–853
34. Kajiwara S (2014) Parameter study of a step-climbing machine for heavy load carriers. J Robot Mechatron 26(3):341–348
35. Ariga A, Yamaguchi T, Hashimoto S (2011) Passively adaptable wall climbing robot in narrow space. J Robot Mechatron 23(6):1055–1065
36. Baishya NJ, Ogai H (2018) Wa-chair: a concept for development of economical stair-climbing wheelchair. In: IOP conference series: materials science and engineering, vol 307, pp 012010
37. Baishya NJ, Ogai H, Bhattacharya B (2019) Design and development of a new active slider crank mechanism based step climbing wheelchair. In: 12th Asian control conference (ASCC), pp 271–276
38. Baishya NJ, Bhattacharya B, Ogai H, Tatsumi K (2021) Analysis and design of a minimalist step climbing robot. App Sci 11, (15):7044. https://doi.org/10.3390/app11157044
39. Mori Y, Katsumura K, Nagase K (2015) Feasibility study of a pair of 2-DOF step-climbing units for a manual wheelchair user. In: 12th international conference on informatics in control, automation and robotics (ICINCO), vol 2, pp 196–201

# 4 Design and Development of a Left Ventricular Assist Device

K. Muralidhar, Niraj Sinha, Pranav R. Joshi, Nikunj Bhagat, Amitabha Bandyopadhyay, Jayandharan R. Rao, and Kantesh Balani

**Abstract**

The importance of building left ventricular assist devices (LVADs) that help the left ventricle pump blood into the aorta is now being acutely felt worldwide. The device is clearly indispensable, serving as a vital and enduring solution for patients afflicted by partial heart failure. Design, development and testing of such devices poses several challenges in view of the tight tolerances to be achieved in terms of weight, volume, power consumption, noise and durability. A few international products that have emerged over the years suffer biocompatibility issues, such as hemolysis and pump thrombosis while increasing chances of stroke and gastrointestinal bleeding. This article covers progress over the past two years at IIT Kanpur and ongoing effort toward building an indigenously engineered LVAD that has its own aspects of innovation and uniqueness. The methodology adopted and benchmarks attained are highlighted. Additionally, there is an immense potential for spin-off technologies. The pump is made of medical grade titanium with a volume small enough to fit within the pericardial space below the human heart. The impeller blades of the centrifugal pump are polished while the volume casing is sintered and support hemocompatibility aspects of the blood-contacting surfaces. The next development targeted for the prototype introduces 3D maglev, where the rotor will entirely be supported magnetically without any physical bearing support to run at high speeds, typically 8000 rpm. It is an important design feature that ensures low noise and low power consumption. On an average, the device will be capable of delivering 5 LPM flow rate at a pressure head of around

K. Muralidhar (✉) · N. Sinha · P. R. Joshi
Department of Mechanical Engineering, Gangwal School of Medical Sciences and Technology, Indian Institute of Technology Kanpur, Kanpur, India
e-mail: kmurli@iitk.ac.in

N. Sinha
e-mail: nsinha@iitk.ac.in

P. R. Joshi
e-mail: jpranavr@iitk.ac.in

N. Bhagat
Departments of Electrical Engineering and Biological Sciences and Bioengineering, Gangwal School of Medical Sciences and Technology, Indian Institute of Technology Kanpur, Kanpur, India
e-mail: nbhagat@iitk.ac.in

A. Bandyopadhyay · J. R. Rao
Department of Biological Sciences and Bioengineering, Gangwal School of Medical Sciences and Technology, Indian Institute of Technology Kanpur, Kanpur, India
e-mail: abandopa@iitk.ac.in

J. R. Rao
e-mail: jrrao@iitk.ac.in

K. Balani
Department of Materials Science and Engineering, Gangwal School of Medical Sciences and Technology, Indian Institute of Technology Kanpur, Kanpur, India
e-mail: kbalani@iitk.ac.in



S. Verma (ed.), *Technology and Innovation in Medical Sciences*, IITK Directions 7,
https://doi.org/10.1007/978-981-96-8606-3_4

100 mm Hg while consuming below 5 W power. The entire device requires development of dedicated electronics for both speed and position control and forms a substantial part of the project. In the ongoing in vitro evaluations with the final device prototype, biocompatibility (cytotoxicity, chemical characterizations) and blood damage profile (RBC damage, platelet activation and infections) are scrutinized by conducting hemolysis loop tests. The data thus generated leads us into animal trials.

**Keywords**

Left ventricular assist device · Pump characteristics · Motor design · Maglev system · Biocompatibility · Hemolysis · In vitro tests

## 4.1 Introduction

Congestive heart failure is said to affect over 64 million people worldwide, with 9–10 million cases in India alone. On one hand, national health data show that barely 10–15 heart transplants happen each year in India. On the other, more than 50,000 people lose their lives annually to heart failure. A significant number of patients are deemed ineligible for a heart transplant owing to factors such as age, weight, and comorbidities and there is a pressing demand for a viable and enduring alternative therapy. The use of left ventricular assist device (LVAD)—A high performance device that helps the left ventricle pump blood into the aorta is an alternative. The use of the device clearly serves as a vital and enduring solution for patients afflicted by heart weakening and failure.

The challenge lies in the fact that all LVADs implanted in India are imported and carry a substantial cost. In view of the considerable cost of the device, as well as that of surgery and hospitalization, obtaining an LVAD remains a feasible choice for only a limited number of individuals. Furthermore, biocompatibility issues, such as hemolysis, thrombosis, stroke, and gastrointestinal bleeding, continue to be associated with the commercially available device, detrimental to the prospects of patient survival.

At the Gangwal School of Medical Science and Technology, a project was launched in late 2021 to address the challenges related to heart ailments and lack of availability of biomedical devices that promote patient well-being. Specifically, the aim was to develop an innovative, indigenously engineered LVAD that excels in performance, comfort, longevity and cost. The goal was to make the implantation of this device accessible to a significantly larger number of individuals experiencing end-stage heart failure. Additionally, the project aimed at developing a device with enhanced hemocompatibility compared to current options, thereby positively influencing treatment outcomes on an international scale. With this ambition, *Mission Hridyantra* commenced in May 2022 with a research group of nine well-qualified individuals of varied expertise, both from academia and the industry, and mentored by a faculty group from the institute. Additionally, several reputed medical doctors from across the country pledged to participate in discussions and provide logistic support.

In the past few years, a self-contained laboratory has been set up while substantial progress has been accomplished in product design and development. We describe this journey, highlight novel aspects, and outline tasks that remain to be completed.

## 4.2 Specifications

The specifications of the LVAD as an implantable pump are laid out here. It is expected to deliver a certain flow rate of blood ($Q$) with a concomitant pressure rise, measured in terms of the head ($H$) of the mercury column. A centrifugal pump design is adopted that can deliver 2–9 LPM of blood for a pressure rise of 60–150 mm Hg [1]. To account for patient-scale variability and the possibility of other disturbances in the device itself, the pump is expected to operate over a range of speeds, possibly from 3000 to 9000 rpm. The pump, driven by a brushless DC motor, runs at a constant rotational speed by design that can be controlled externally through an electronic circuit. The device is also expected to provide support for a weakened heart whose left ventricle is still partially functional and provides the required pulsatility to the flow delivered in the human body.

Other specifications that characterize the device are as follows: Material of construction mainly medical grade titanium alloy for the pump and silicon steel for the motor; a weight below 250 g; volume of 100 ml or smaller; an operational speed up to 10,000 rpm; a noise level of <2 dB; a power consumption of <5 W; longevity ~5 years; and battery-operated with a drive line connected to the pump.

The percentage of the electrical power input that gets converted to a pressure rise may be of the order of 5–10% over a range of rpm and flow rates. A significant part of the input is required to overcome internal friction in the liquid medium and copper losses in the electrical windings. Mechanical losses in the bearings are expected to be of the order 5%.

The device is expected to be safe against hemolysis of blood and thrombus formation, calling for specialized characteristics of the blood-contacting surfaces. Keeping the power consumption and noise level low demands eliminating metal-to-metal contact, particularly at bearings. A viable substitute in the form of a full magnetically levitated arrangement is being introduced.

Considerable progress has been achieved in the past two years. The device has undergone multiple laboratory-scale trials. It has achieved geometric finality as well as hydromechanical and electrical functionalities [2]. While in vitro tests of the running device are in progress, in vivo studies in the form of animal trials are close to being conducted.

## 4.3 Pathway of Progress

The configuration of the LVAD under development is shown as an exploded view in Fig. 4.1.

During the design and development process, several versions of the device were prepared. These versions underwent careful modifications to achieve the required specifications and performance. The first prototype, version 1.1 of the device was fabricated using PMMA material (polymethyl methacrylate) by CNC machining. Among the possible designs of impellers shown in Fig. 4.2 (first row), version 1.1 has four impellers, involves an optimized blood flow path and the necessary electronics to run the motor at the required flow rate. Version 1.2 of the device was prepared with metallic parts. The inflow cannula, outer body, volute casing and outflow cannula were fabricated in aluminum alloy 6061 using CNC machining available in the Medtech Center of the institute. A sample pressure head (mm of Hg) versus flow rate (l pm) graph is also shown in Fig. 4.2 (second row). Extensive tests show that the performance of version 1.1 is already close to the specifications of commercially available devices.

The third version of the device was fabricated using medical grade titanium alloy and was equipped with an indigenously made motor and electronics. The key feature of version 1.3 is that it is practically noise-free and has minimal heat generation even at high rotational speeds and flow rate.

The present version 1.4 is of medical grade titanium alloy and works on partial (passive) maglev principle. In this version, the rotor is supported by only a pivot point to maintain stability of its axis during rotation and is an improvement over the conventional shafted support where friction levels are higher. The pivot is located within ruby bearings where surface friction is low and thermal conductivity is high. The second factor is useful in keeping temperature build-up at permissible levels. A key aspect of version 1.4 is biocompatibility. The blood-contacting surfaces of the device are modified to specific values of

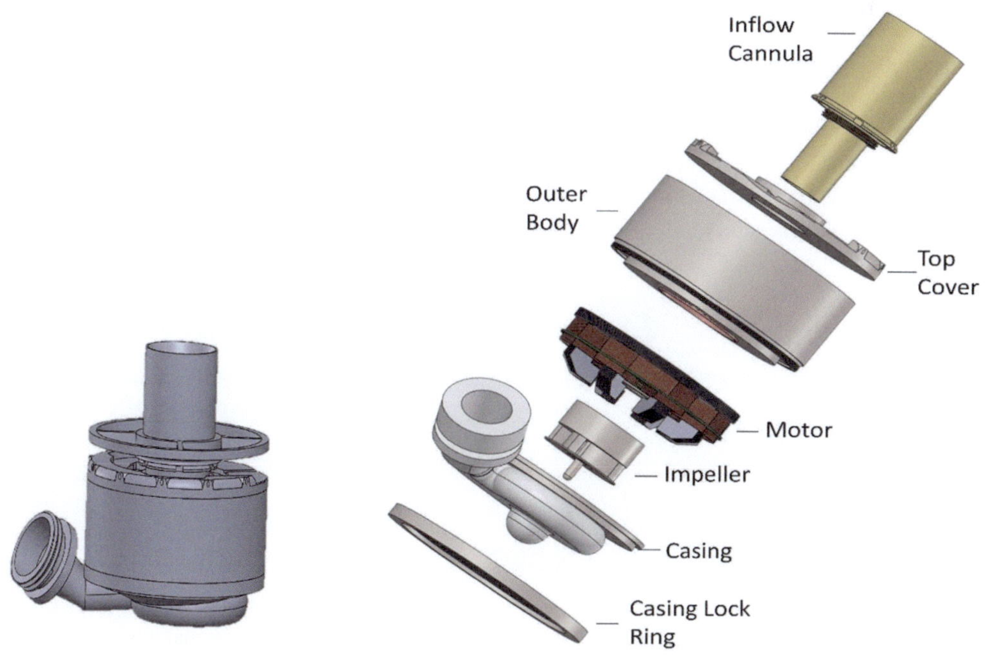


**Fig. 4.1** Exploded view (right) of a left ventricular assist device showing the pump-motor assembly (left). The impeller also carries the permanent magnet that driven by the motor

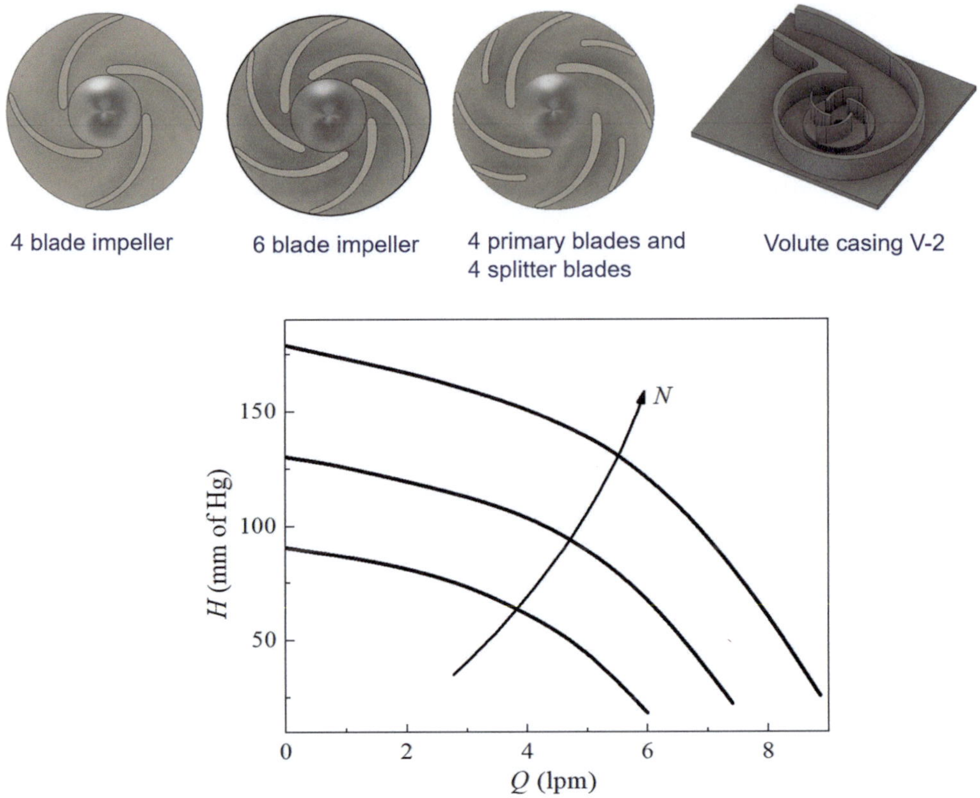


**Fig. 4.2** (First row) Impeller designs considered for the blood pump along with the volute casing; (second row) Head ($H$)-flow ($Q$) characteristics at various impeller speeds ($N$, rpm = 4000–6000) of a typical centrifugal pump of the type used in LVADs; the data shown in the two axes correspond to factory-manufactured pumps while the laboratory-fabricated version exceeds these expectations. A prototype will typically operate at $Q = 5$ lpm and $H = 100$ mm Hg

roughness, porosity, wettability, and surface morphology. These provide controlled tissue growth, ultimately reducing crucial adverse events, including pump thrombosis, hemolysis, and stroke. In vitro tests of the developed surfaces going all the way to device prototype are being performed using fresh human blood in the hemolysis test loop established within the laboratory.

A pathline of technology development of the LVAD over the past two years described above is summarized in Fig. 4.3.

The next development (version 1.5) that will take the device toward an implantable version is three-dimensional magnetic levitation (*maglev*), where the rotor will be supported magnetically without any physical support over the range of rotational speeds of interest. The improved design is expected to show a significant reduction in power consumption along with low noise levels. A rechargeable battery pack attached to the device through a controller unit with display and alarms should be adequate for support.

Versions 1.4 and 1.5 are presently being subjected to laboratory-scale in vitro tests with human blood from a blood bank with the following perspectives:

*Biocompatibility*: Tests here include rigorous screening of the bare and sintered titanium surfaces for cytotoxicity and comprehensive chemical characterization. Ensuring that the choice of the device material does not induce harmful effects on cells is crucial to its safety and effectiveness in a clinical setting.

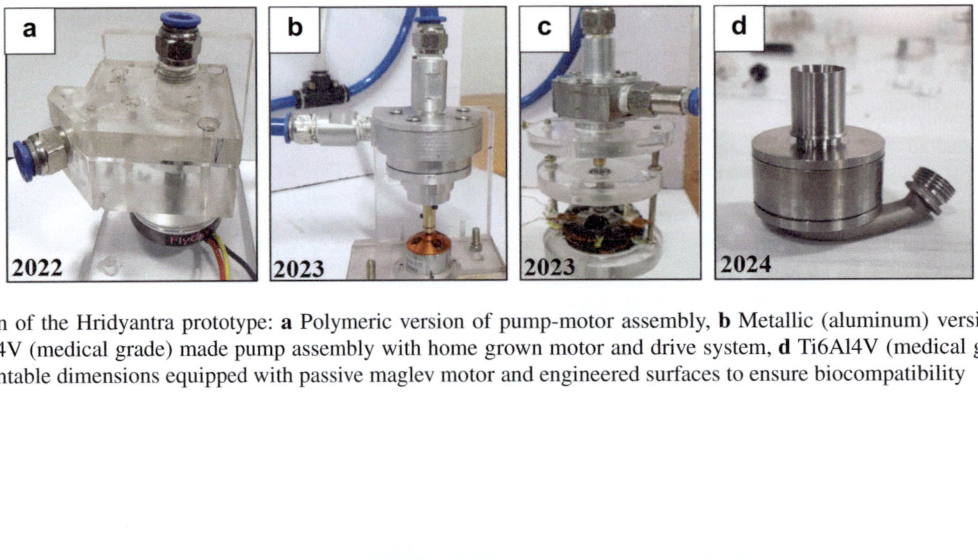


**Fig. 4.3** Evolution of the Hridyantra prototype: **a** Polymeric version of pump-motor assembly, **b** Metallic (aluminum) version of pump-motor assembly, **c** Ti6Al4V (medical grade) made pump assembly with home grown motor and drive system, **d** Ti6Al4V (medical grade) made LVAD assembly of implantable dimensions equipped with passive maglev motor and engineered surfaces to ensure biocompatibility

*Blood Damage Profile*: Tests evaluate how the device interacts with blood components, focusing on the extent of damage to red blood cells (RBCs), activation of platelets, and risks of infection. These factors are crucial for determining the ability of the device to maintain blood health during operation.

Once a satisfactory outcome is achieved from in vitro assessments, it may be concluded that the device meets the safety and performance thresholds as stipulated in ISO and ASTM standards and reports available in the literature. Device screening will then proceed to animal trials. This progression to implantation in animals is essential for validating the device functionality and safety in a physiological environment, paving way to clinical applications.

## 4.4 Maglev Technology for Contactless Bearings

Magnetic levitation (namely, *maglev*) leads to a contactless bearing in the sense that it prevents metal to metal contact at the motor-pump coupling and reduces frictional forces arising from relative motion between the shaft and bearing [3]. Moreover, by avoiding metal-to-metal contact the current required to drive the rotor reduces significantly, which reduces power losses, and heat dissipated and increases life of the battery and that of the device. In LVAD, the central idea is to create a magnetic field using electromagnets that will position the shaft away from the solid walls, during its continuous operation. The feedback signals to the electromagnets are generated using Hall-effect sensors mounted on the motor body. In the implementation adopted in design, axial positioning and tilt correction are achieved using a static magnetic field (passive levitation) while the radial position is corrected by the varying magnetic field (active levitation) using Hall-effect sensors. The feedback electronics are mounted on the body of the motor. A cross-sectional view of the motor with a built-in maglev arrangement is shown in Fig. 4.4.

## 4.5 Extracorporeal Device

The design being finalized in the Hridyantra project is an implantable LVAD that will work in conjunction with a partially weakened human heart. Such a device requires a variety of stringent conditions to be fulfilled to ensure the comfort of the patient on a time scale of several years while ensuring acceptable device performance itself. These conditionalities are less severe if the device is placed outside the human body though joined to the human heart via suitably designed cannulae. Since it is not implanted, the device can be larger, have additional features in terms of electronic controls and use materials in the exterior that are not necessarily hemocompatible and can be tailored to a variety of body types. If the device is required only in the short run, say a few months, titanium may be substituted by polycarbonate and the fabrication cost would be greatly reduced. Surface coatings such as heparin should be adequate as an anti-coagulant. The device may use the maglev approach

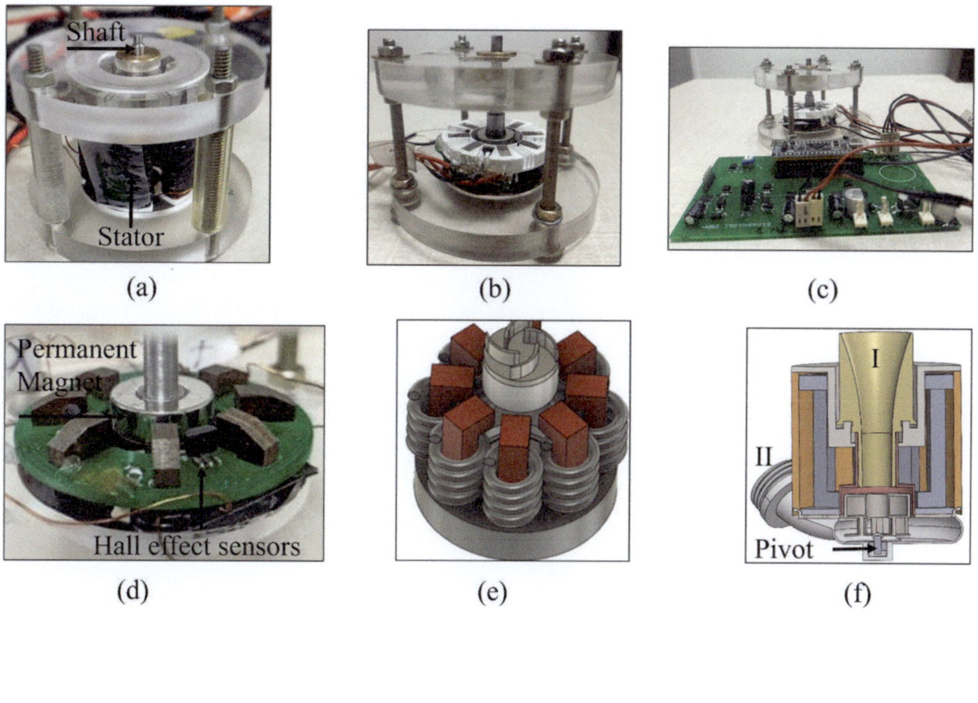


**Fig. 4.4** Layout of a BLDC motor: **a** Prototype of an 8-limb shafted motor with axial levitation. **b** A smaller-sized shafted motor. **c** A motor along with a separate drive PCB. **d** A PCB for the Hall effect sensors on the motor. **e** Schematic of a magnetically levitating rotor/ impeller on an 8-limb motor design. **f** Schematic of a motor and pump assembly with an axially levitating pivoted rotor/ impeller (I-inflow cannula, II-outflow cannula)

merely to reduce friction but complete flotation of the motor shaft in the bearing may not be required. Such a simplified device, called an extracorporeal device, will restrict human mobility but has considerable applications. It is often called a bridge-to-therapy route as opposed to the original LVAD, which is an example of destination therapy. The ongoing project is aimed at building LVADs although extracorporeal devices will emerge as spin-off technologies and widen the product base of the initiative. Version 1.3 described earlier is an example of an extracorporeal device although larger ones can be readily designed.

## 4.6 Testbed

To an extent, the performance characteristics of the device can be simulated using analysis software for fluid dynamics, structural mechanics, and electromagnetics. It is, however, not a substitute for a physical platform where the device can be placed and tested for pressure head—flow rate (*H-Q*) characteristics at various rotational speeds [4]. Individual blade designs can thus be studied in an experimental apparatus while evaluating the possibility of a higher number of blades, split blades, and volute casing geometry. The test bed is also the right platform to study the endurance of the device over a timeframe of hours to days to weeks. The test bed will require sensors for measuring flow rate, pressure head, rotational speed, torque, noise levels, current drawn and voltage supplied. In a real-life context, these quantities are time-dependent; the time series data thus generated will be stored in a computer using a data acquisition system.

In a human body, an LVAD is attached to the heart and the pump works against the pulsations in pressure and flow created by the rhythmic movement of the ventricle. The load on the motor is thus, time-dependent and the electronic circuits that keep the motor speed constant need to be designed against this variability of the external load. The pulsatility of the heart can be factored in the test bed by creating a heart simulator where pulsations in pressure can be created by a variable stroke reciprocating pump, often called a pulse duplicator. The resulting layout is also called a mock circulatory loop. A human heart analog developed in the ongoing project to which the LVAD is connected during tests is shown in Fig. 4.5.

## 4.7 Modeling and Simulation

Mathematical modeling and computer simulation offer a convenient route to ideate product design, analyze performance and optimize parameters in a relatively short time and low cost. In the LVAD context, the pump performance can be evaluated as a function of rotational speed for various blade designs. The simulator will have to account for the principles of hydrodynamics, three-dimensional geometry of the flow space, smoothness and roughness of various surfaces, and blood rheology. The number of parameters that should be varied to achieve peak performance is enormous; for example, the number of blades, blade thickness, blade angles, inner and outer diameters, and others (first row of Fig. 4.2). Numerically determined flow patterns for a centrifugal pump are shown in Fig. 4.6.

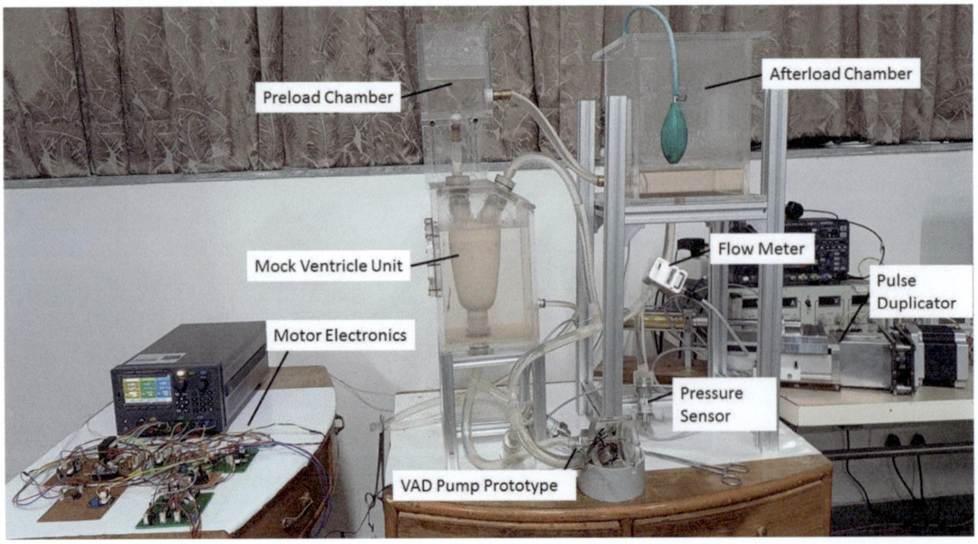


**Fig. 4.5** Photograph of a test bed in which LVAD designs can be introduced to check for their performance. A heart simulator (labeled *mock ventricle unit*) creates pressure pulses over the device analogous to the human heart

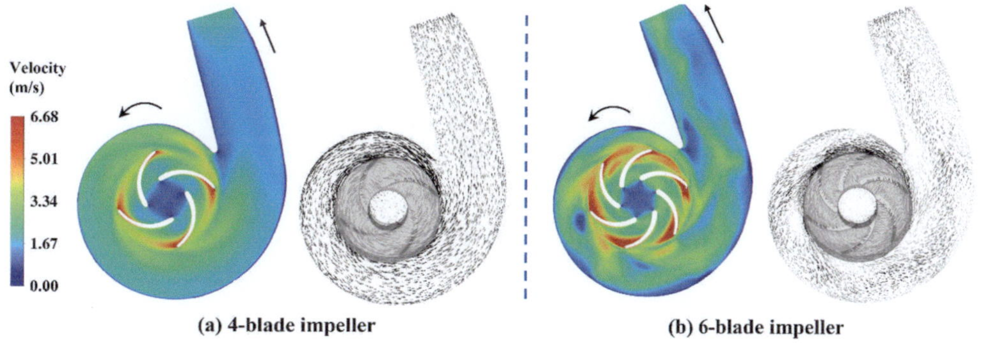


**Fig. 4.6** Velocity contours and vectors around impellers rotating at 7000 rpm providing a flow rate of 5.7 LPM. **a** 4-blade (head = 134.4 mm Hg) and **b** 6-blade impeller (head = 118.3 mm Hg). Velocities in the central portion are in the rotating frame of reference while, beyond the impeller, velocities are in an inertial frame of reference

For the electrical drive, an equally large number of parameters can be imagined, for example, the number of poles, coil wire diameter and number of turns, and parameters of the feedback circuit related to position and speed control. It is unthinkable that these many parameters are varied one at a time in an experimental framework. Simulations are a convenient alternative that also lay the ground rules for optimization, namely, the set of values of parameters that will, in a predefined sense, deliver peak performance. It may be pointed out that device optimization can be effectively performed by constructing a *digital twin*, namely, a virtual representation of the functioning device, in a cost-effective manner.

## 4.8 Hemolysis and Thrombosis

The damage to red blood corpuscles during their passage through the pump is called hemolysis. A variety of methods are available to quantify hemolysis although the hemolysis index (HI) is one of them that is often used. The higher the index, the higher the damage. Under ideal conditions, pump hemolysis should be limited such that the body has a chance to rejuvenate itself continuously over the concerned period of time. The origin of hemolysis is shear stress within the flowing medium and the residence time of RBCs in regions of high shear stress. It has a numerical value that is the product of these two factors. It reaches a peak at the impeller blades where surface speeds, and hence, shear stresses, are very high. Shear stresses are lower when the impeller blades are highly polished and serve as a means to control hemolysis. Mathematical models can predict hemolysis index distribution and identify local regions where it is high. The design can be suitably refined in these zones of high risk. Simulated distributions of HI around the impeller blades of the centrifugal pump of the LVAD are shown in Fig. 4.7.

Thrombosis relates to clot formation in the pump and is often seen in regions of lower speeds and recirculation zones, for example, the flow passage in the volute casing. Such deposits may detach from the wall at later times and enter the main bloodstream. This possibility can be fatal to the patient and should be avoided at all costs. Mathematical models of thrombus formation are also available and the possibility of formation of deposit can be systematically investigated. A precautionary

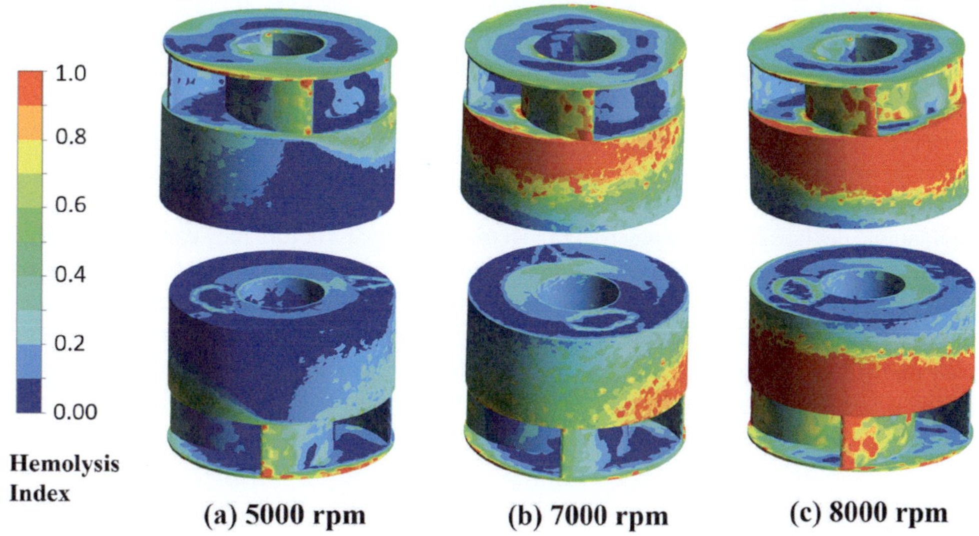


**Fig. 4.7** Blood damage quantified by the hemolysis index for unit inflow (LPM) compared at rotational speeds of **a** 5000, **b** 7000, and **c** 8000 rpm for a 4-blade impeller. The first and the second rows show two views of the pump. Higher blood damage is clearly revealed as red patches at higher rotational speeds

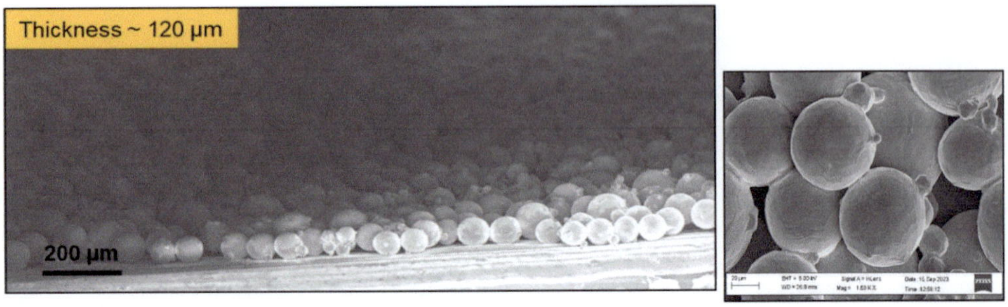


**Fig. 4.8** A close-up view of a titanium substrate with titanium powder sintering along with an image from FESEM (right)

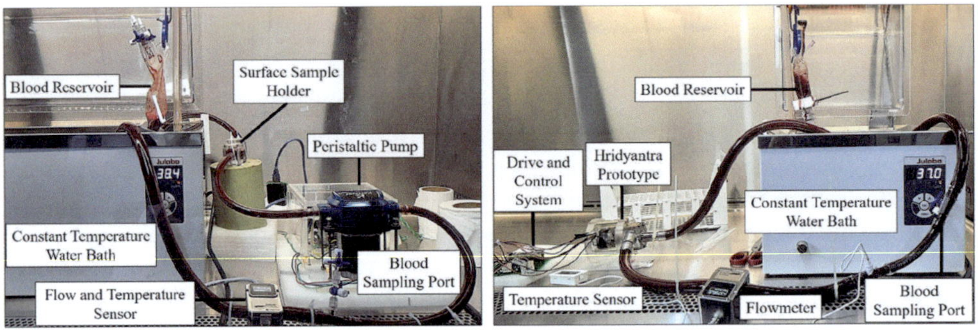


**Fig. 4.9** Photographs of a hemolysis loop set-up **as per ASTM 1841–19 standard** with a peristaltic pump for hemocompatibility surface testing (left) and for the device itself (right) in the Hridyantra laboratory

alternative is to sinter the stationary blood contacting surfaces with multiple layers of powdered titanium. Such surfaces encourage and stabilize the formation of intima, a layer that is found in the blood vessels of the human body. In this respect, the pathway with the pump becomes similar to the artery and delays any possibility of clotting. A close-up view of a sintered surface is shown in Fig. 4.8.

Protection against hemolysis and thrombosis must be guaranteed from in vitro tests even before animal trials [5, 6]. The protocol for such in vitro tests is laid out in ISO and ASTM standards. A photograph of a hemolysis loop set up within the Hridyantra laboratory is shown in Fig. 4.9. The loop closely mimics the actual physiological environment and is capable of creating flow rates and temperature over a range, as required to accurately assess the adverse impact of the device on blood cells and plasma proteins. During these trials, the blood damage profile is evaluated by hemolysis assays, complete blood counts, platelet activation evaluation, and von Willebrand factor collagen binding assessment, measures that are crucial for identifying potential risks of stroke, infection, bleeding, and thrombus formation. Tests such as platelet activation evaluation and von Willebrand factor collagen binding assessment are specialized and require sophisticated equipment. The normalized HI is a reliable indicator of device suitability for implantation and depends on flow parameters, test duration and changes in the plasma-free hemoglobin that may increase from 20 to 100 mg/dl over a 6–8 h period. The HI is a direct measure of RBC damage. Whole blood samples are drawn from the hemolysis loop at pre-determined intervals to quantify the hemoglobin suspended in blood plasma from the damaged RBCs. Here, the free hemoglobin concentration in plasma is measured with a spectrophotometer that examines the ultra-violet absorptance of the plasma samples.

## 4.9 Animal Trials

Implantable devices require extensive clinical trials in humans before they can be accepted for routine medical surgery. A step before clinical trials is animal trials where the device developed is implanted in select animals for varying time intervals. Pigs are acceptable for implantation of a few hours; sheep may be selected for a few days while calves may be tested for a period of several months. Animals are first stabilized in the operation theater in a few hours. They are later freed with the battery pack mounted as a pouch on their body. Implanted animals will be in a cohort and their behavior such as appetite, mood, and bowel movement remotely monitored using CCTV cameras. Animal implantation is conducted by veterinary surgeons in select government-approved laboratories.

## 4.10 Infrastructure Support

Rolling out biomedical products, specifically those based on biomechanical pumps requires an extensive and certified manufacturing base. Equipment include 5-axis CNC machines, metal and polymer 3D printers, surface finishing and electropolishing setups, vacuum sintering furnaces, and optical and surface characterization facilities. A sophisticated electrical fabrication laboratory for building control circuits and the associated electronics, and sensors and data acquisition arrangement will have to be developed. A reasonably clean room (class 1000) for in vitro tests related to blood-surface interactions and a hemolysis loop has to be created. The device will be tuned for each patient and will require a battery pack along with a console as control and processing unit. A device such as an LVAD is designed to run for years of uninterrupted operation and hence, alignment and assembly-related fixtures have to be put in place. Design alternatives can be tested via simulation, and an effective computing environment with analysis software is essential. Overall, the initiative calls for substantial and long-term investment in space, hardware, and trained manpower.

## 4.11 Future Prospects

Cardiovascular devices, both hardware and software, have long development cycles and require extensive animal and human testing before use. As a result, most of these are imported, becoming costly and beyond the reach of the local population. The productization of a blood pump and its variants can be accelerated by leveraging recent advances in artificial intelligence and digital twin technologies, ultimately enabling in silico (or, computational) *cardiology*. The digital twins approach helps optimize, as well as customize, designs on an acceptable time frame and a lower cost.

The LVAD device that runs on 3D maglev technology on contactless bearings at high speeds with the required flow rate and pressure rise is a forerunner of a *total artificial heart* (TAH). This expectation follows from the design of a TAH which has a left and right ventricle mounted on a common shaft with shared electronics and control strategy. The development of a total artificial heart is poised to revolutionize Indian healthcare, showcasing not only technological strength but also making a substantial contribution to the nation's economy. Specifically, the trajectory involving the development of an LVAD and a cardiovascular digital twin, in the pursuit of a total artificial heart represents a significant leap forward for healthcare in India.

**Acknowledgements** This article was prepared with technical inputs from Mandeep Singh, Supriya Das, Rushit Bhanderi, Akshay Namdeo, Vinay Tripathi, and Mohammad Owais. The Hridyantra project receives extensive support in manufacturing, fabrication, and assembly from Phool Chand Gond, H.P. Sharma, and Manoj Sharma. Financial support from Class of 1976; Mr. N.R. Narayana Murthy and Mrs. Sudha Murthy, Bangalore; Vacmet, Agra; Portescap, Mumbai; and ICMR, New Delhi is deeply appreciated. Technical discussions with doctors from Narayana Health, Bangalore, particularly Dr(s) Devi Shetty and Julius Punnen; SGPGI, Lucknow; and Palamur Biosciences Hyderabad have been essential for conducting this project. Dr. Lubna Khan and her team from GSVM Medical College, Kanpur provided assistance in securing human blood from the blood bank. Finally, the authors are grateful to IIT Kanpur for providing space, administrative support, a wide range of dedicated machinery and characterization facilities, and financial support when required.

## References

1. Yazdanpanah-Ardakani K, Niroomand-Oscuii H, Sahebi-Kuzeh Kanan R, Shokri N (2024) Optimization of a centrifugal blood pump designed using an industrial method through experimental and numerical study. Sci Rep 14(1):7443
2. Mihalj M, Heinisch PP, Schober P, Wieser M, Martinelli M, de By TM, Reineke D (2022) Third-generation continuous-flow left ventricular assist devices: a comparative outcome analysis by device type. ESC Hear Fail 9(5):3469–3482
3. Schmitto JD, Shaw S, Garbade J, Gustafsson F, Morshuis M, Zimpfer D, Saeed D (2024) Fully magnetically centrifugal left ventricular assist device and long-term outcomes: the ELEVATE registry. Eur Heart J 45(8):613–625
4. Xu KW, Gao Q, Wan M, Zhang K (2023) Mock circulatory loop applications for testing cardiovascular assist devices and in vitro studies. Front Physiol 14:1175919
5. He W, Butcher JT, Rowlands GW, Antaki JF (2023) Biological response to sintered titanium in left ventricular assist devices: pseudoneointima, neointima, and pannus. ASAIO J 69(1):1–10
6. Zayat R, Moza A, Grottke O, Grzanna T, Fechter T, Motomura T, Bleilevens C (2019) In vitro comparison of the hemocompatibility of two centrifugal left ventricular assist devices. J Thorac Cardiovasc Surg 157(2):591–599

# 5 Development of Percutaneous Ventricular Assist Devices

Pranav Joshi, Niraj Sinha, Rakesh Kumar, Nikunj Bhagat, B. V. Rathish Kumar, and K. Muralidhar

**Abstract**

Percutaneous ventricular assist devices (pVADs) are non-implantable miniature blood pumps that can be used during cardiac recovery and high-risk coronary interventions. Despite the high prevalence of cardiovascular diseases, the use of such devices in India has been limited due to their prohibitively high cost, largely a result of the absence of indigenous manufacturers. In response to this situation, a project has been initiated under the Gangwal School of Medical Science and Technology that aims to leverage the expertise and infrastructure available at IIT Kanpur to develop a high-end pVAD that will not only be available to a substantially greater section of the population and improve clinical outcomes but also contribute to the development of a medical device manufacturing ecosystem in the country.

**Keywords**

pVAD · Blood pump · Micromotor · Guidewire · Catheter · Hemolysis · *H-Q* characteristics

## 5.1 Background

Percutaneous ventricle assist devices (pVADs) are non-implantable temporary-support devices that are deployed during cardiac recovery following acute cardiac conditions such as cardiogenic shock (inability of the heart to pump enough blood) and acute myocardial infarction (heart attack) with cardiogenic shock. Such a device, which has a blood pump as its primary component, aids the recovery of the heart by decreasing the pumping load on the heart and increasing blood perfusion in the coronary arteries by lowering the pressure in the ventricle. The device can also be used for high-risk percutaneous coronary interventions (in which it can provide support if the heart fails to pump blood) and as a 'bridge to transplant' for a patient waiting for a heart transplant. Since cardiovascular diseases (CVDs) have become the leading cause of mortality in India contributing to about 25% of the total deaths [1], the need for such devices is evident. However, these devices suffer from excessive blood damage [2] and are expensive (costing approximately INR 25 lakh in India). Also, there are no indigenous manufacturers in the country. In response, the current project was started a year ago as one of the flagship projects of the

P. Joshi (✉) · N. Sinha · K. Muralidhar
Department of Mechanical Engineering, Indian Institute of Technology Kanpur, Kanpur, India
e-mail: jpranavr@iitk.ac.in

R. Kumar
Department of Aerospace Engineering, Indian Institute of Technology Kanpur, Kanpur, India

N. Bhagat
Department of Electrical Engineering, Indian Institute of Technology Kanpur, Kanpur, India

Department of Biological Sciences and Bioengineering, Indian Institute of Technology Kanpur, Kanpur, India

B. V. Rathish Kumar
Department of Mathematics and Statistics, Indian Institute of Technology Kanpur, Kanpur, India


S. Verma (ed.), *Technology and Innovation in Medical Sciences*, IITK Directions 7,
https://doi.org/10.1007/978-981-96-8606-3_5

Gangwal School of Medical Science and Technology. It aims to leverage the technical expertise and the infrastructure available at IIT Kanpur to develop a high-end percutaneous VAD that will be superior to the market-available devices, thus improving patient treatment outcomes, be affordably priced so that it will be made available to a larger section of the population, and provide a boost to medical device manufacturing in the country.

Percutaneous VADs come in various configurations, however, they are catheter-based devices and hence do not need major surgical interventions. The version being pursued by our team consists of a miniaturized blood pump that delivers blood from a ventricle (left or right) to the corresponding artery at the desired flow rate and pressure. The pump may be driven by an extracorporeal (outside the human body) electric motor or a miniaturized electric motor integrated with the pump at one end of a catheter. The catheter is introduced into the arterial system through, e.g., the femoral artery, and maneuvered so that the blood pump is positioned in proximity to the appropriate valve at the outlet of the concerned ventricle. A pVAD comprises multiple components such as catheters and guidewires, a miniaturized blood pump, a miniaturized high-speed motor, and high-end control electronics. The targeted device will have the following specifications: pump flow output of 2.5–3.0 lit/min at a pressure rise of 80–100 mm Hg, and a small cross-section of 4 mm diameter. The device will be optimized for low noise, low power consumption, and ease of deployment. In the following sections, the details of the various subsystems will be discussed, along with the challenges in their development and the progress made so far.

## 5.2 Blood Pump

At the heart of the pVAD is a blood pump driven by an electric motor. The motor can be either embedded inside the catheter or can be extracorporeal. In the former case, the motor is miniaturized and integrated with the pump, while in the latter case, although there is no restriction on the motor size, the motor needs to be connected to the pump using a flexible cable routed through the catheter that can transmit torque at very high rotation speeds. The pump itself consists of an impeller (also called the rotor), which is housed in a circular casing. The requirements of flow, pressure rise, and space constraints (percutaneous introduction) dictate the use of an axial pump, i.e., one in which the inflow and outflow of the fluid are parallel to the rotation axis. A model of such a pump is shown in Fig. 5.1a, in which the catheter forms a cylindrical casing around the impeller. The impeller is supported at its two ends by low-friction bearings. The function of the impeller is to provide the required flow rate of blood at sufficient pressure, and its performance is characterized in the form of $H$-$Q$ curves, where $H$ is the pressure rise through the pump measured in terms of the height (in mm) of the mercury column and $Q$ is the flow rate in lit/min.

Developing a small-scale blood pump imposes several challenges. The miniature impeller should be fabricated using blood-compatible materials. Accuracy has to be maintained at small scales and high-performance bearings have to be designed for smooth operation and minimum heating. The contact of the blood with the motor (if integrated into the catheter) and its entry into the tiny spaces between rotating and stationary parts have to be avoided, and tight clearances between the rotor and the casing have to be managed to minimize blood damage while ensuring low noise, vibration, and extended operational life.

Impellers of various shapes have been designed and tested by our team for their $H$-$Q$ characteristics to arrive at an optimum design. An impeller made from a biocompatible polymer using 3D printing is shown in Fig. 5.1b and c. The blade designs are tested using both experiments and numerical simulations. To characterize the impellers experimentally, a testbed (see Fig. 5.2a) has been developed that enables the measurement of the flow rate and the pressure rise through the pump at various rotor speeds. The testbed employs an axial pump housed in a larger conduit, an arrangement that closely mimics the position of the pVAD pump in the human aorta during deployment (see Fig. 5.2b). The pump is currently powered by a 'macro' motor (of size around 40 mm, see next section) and will be integrated with the miniaturized electric motor when the latter is ready. Sample $H$-$Q$ curves recorded using blood-mimicking fluid are presented in Fig. 5.2c and show that the impeller design can be tweaked to obtain a more desirable (flatter) $H$-$Q$ curve that prevents excessive suction inside the ventricle at low flow rates. Further development will involve fine-tuning the impeller design, inclusion of high-performance bearings,

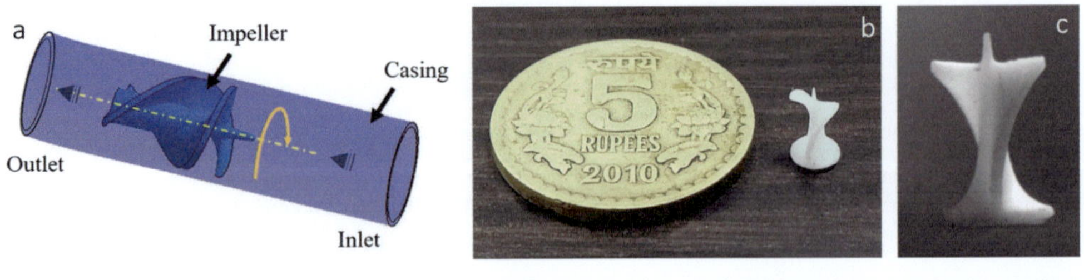


**Fig. 5.1** **a** Schematic of an axial pump, **b** a sample 3D printed impeller, **c** zoomed view of the impeller

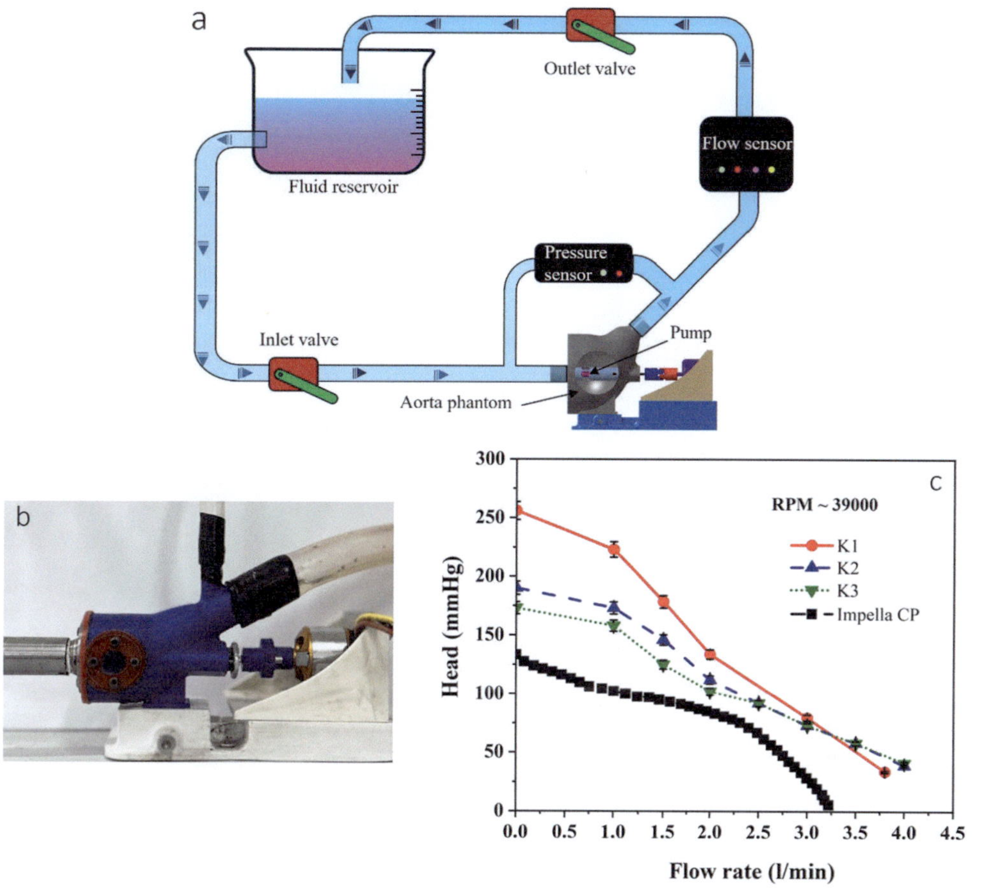


**Fig. 5.2** **a** Schematic of the testbed, **b** test configuration incorporating an axial pump inside an aorta phantom, **c** $H$-$Q$ characteristics for sample impellers at 39,000 RPM. The data for Impella CP (commercially available pVAD from Abiomed Inc.) has been obtained from [3]

increasing manufacturing precision, incorporating a purge system, and testing with human blood. While the current testbed only enables performance measurement under steady-state operation, an advanced testbed is being assembled that will enable pump performance assessment under physiologically relevant unsteady operating conditions.

Our team has also used computational fluid dynamics (CFD) simulations to complement the experimental data. CFD simulations are a powerful tool to assess device performance and compare various designs to arrive at an optimum one. In addition to corroborating $H$-$Q$ data from experiments, CFD simulations are valuable in assessing the flow patterns and their impact on the hemocompatibility of various designs. In the present context, hemolysis and thrombosis are the two important effects that depend on the details of the flow field. Hemolysis is the rupture of blood cells and is dependent on the stress levels the cells are exposed to and the exposure time. Miniature axial pumps, owing to their small size, thin gaps, and high speed, are more prone to hemolysis. Consequently, special attention needs to be paid to hemolysis in their design. The distribution of shear stress on the solid surfaces (Fig. 5.3a) and the volume fraction of the fluid in the device exposed to various stress levels (Fig. 5.3b), for example, can provide a qualitative comparison among different designs for their potential for hemolysis. Lower levels of wall shear and a smaller fraction of fluid volume exposed to high shear auger well for blood health. While more quantitative ways of estimating hemolysis are being implemented, the same will be extended for unsteady pump operation. The analysis of flow patterns to assess the potential for thrombosis, i.e., blood coagulation, is also being carried out.

## 5.3 Motor and Electronics

The electric motor is the prime mover for the blood pump. As indicated earlier, the motor can either be an extracorporeal one provided with a thin cable that transmits torque to the pump, or a miniature motor integrated with the pump. Both versions are being pursued by our team. A brushless direct current (BLDC) motor has been selected for the application since such a configuration can provide a higher torque in a compact size in comparison to other arrangements. A BLDC motor consists of a rotor housing a permanent magnet, which is placed in a magnetic field generated by several electromagnets. The

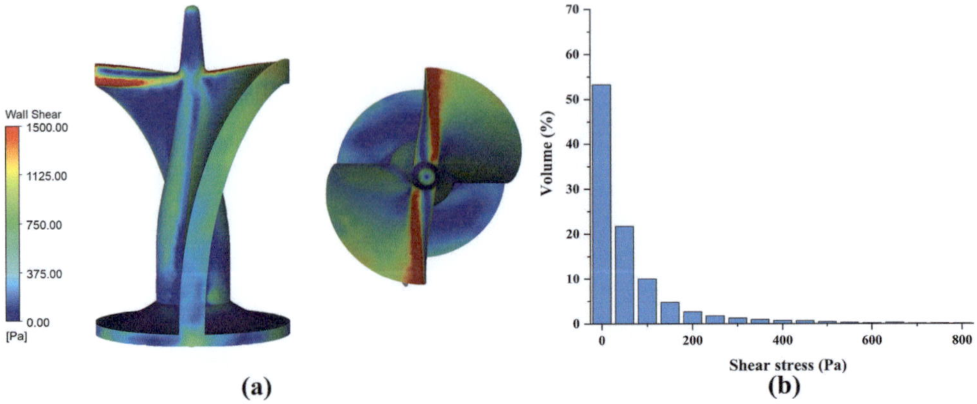


**Fig. 5.3** **a** Distribution of shear stress on the surface of the impeller and **b** histogram of shear stress levels in the fluid volume within the pump for a sample impeller running at 46,000 RPM

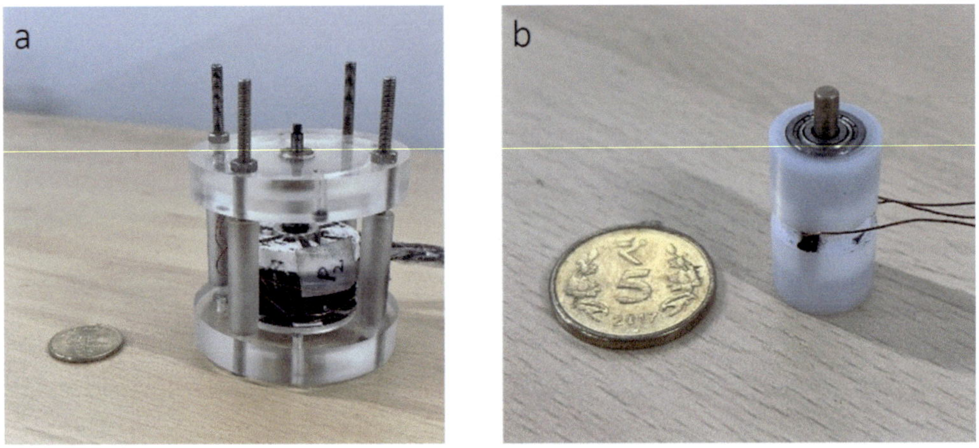


**Fig. 5.4** **a** Macro and **b** mini motors

electromagnets typically consist of current-carrying conductors wound around metallic cores and are energized in precise sequence so that a rotating magnetic field is produced that makes the rotor turn. The control circuit detects the rotor position and energizes the required electromagnets with the appropriate voltage levels to control the rotor speed and provide the torque required for a particular application.

The integrated motor design, due to its small size, presents numerous challenges. The motor has to be miniaturized (micromotor) with diameter smaller than 4 mm. Small but powerful magnets must be housed in the rotor, the windings that generate the magnetic fields have to be accommodated in the narrow annular region between the rotor and the casing, unconventional core (or coreless) designs as well as windings may have to be implemented, miniature sensors have to be incorporated to detect rotor position, and the motor has to be designed for minimum heat generation, low noise, and continuous operation for weeks.

Our team has adopted the approach of developing a medium-sized motor (see Fig. 5.4a) with its associated control electronics and algorithms, and then decreasing its size in successive iterations and modifying the electronics as needed. Accordingly, a 'macro' motor approximately 40 mm in diameter and 40 mm in length has been developed. Control circuits incorporating sensors to detect rotor position and control algorithms have been designed and implemented. Following a similar approach, the size has been reduced to develop the minimotor with an external diameter of 12 mm and a length of 20 mm (Fig. 5.4b). Currently, the control electronics of the minimotor is being optimized to run the motor at speeds up to 20,000 rpm. Concept designs for the micromotor of 4 mm diameter and speed up to 50,000 rpm are being worked on with accompanying numerical simulations to test the feasibility of such designs.

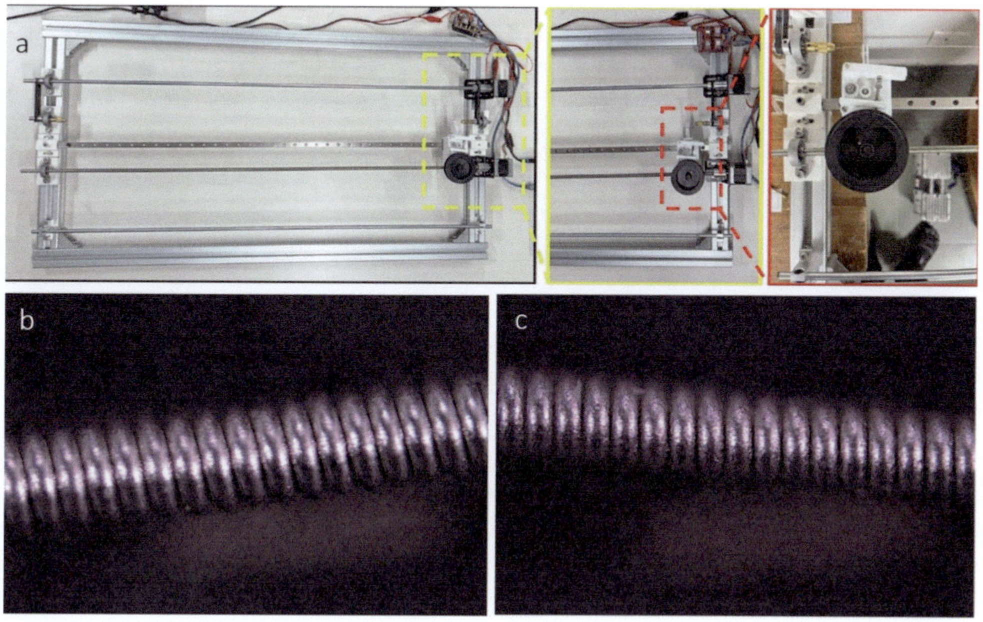


**Fig. 5.5** **a** Guidewire coiling machine, **b** a 400-micron guidewire, and **c** the same guidewire coated with a hemophobic coating

## 5.4 Guidewires and Catheters

Guidewires and catheters are the linchpins of all catheterization procedures such as angiography, intra-vascular lithotripsy, intravascular OCT (optical coherence tomography) imaging, stent delivery, thrombus aspiration, and administration of devices such as intra-aortic balloon pumps. In the context of pVAD, a guidewire is first inserted into the arterial network of the patient and maneuvered such that its distal end rests inside the left ventricle. Following that, a catheter that carries the blood pump near its distal end is introduced into the blood vessel. The catheter is slid over the guidewire until the blood pump is positioned appropriately in relation to the aortic valve with the guidewire acting as a guiding rail for translating the catheter.

A guidewire is a metallic wire with a diameter between 0.3 and 2 mm, depending on the application. It generally consists of a 'core' with another wire coiled around it. The former imparts stiffness to the guidewire while the latter prevents kinking and provides the necessary flexibility. Depending on the application, the combination of the core and coiling wires can also be covered with a coating that provides the guidewire with hemophilic or hemophobic properties. The distal region of the guidewire may possess different shapes and physical properties, along with a specialized tip, to enable efficient maneuvering of the guidewire and patient safety. A guidewire must have properties such as hemocompatibility, trackability to be able to be maneuvered around tortuous blood vessels, radiopacity to be monitored using radio imaging, low tip load to ensure that the wire bends at its tip when pushed hard instead of puncturing a blood vessel, and pushability and tortuosity, respectively, so that any pushing force and torque applied at its proximal end are appropriately transferred to its distal tip.

To ensure the above properties, wires of appropriate material and size have been selected. A wire coiling machine has been built in-house (see Fig. 5.5a) to wind the coiling wire over the core. The machine can use wires of various materials and sizes, and also provide a user-selectable pitch (spacing between successive turns of the coiling wire). A microscope image of a guidewire wound in the lab is shown in Fig. 5.5b. The tip of the guidewire is treated to form a hemispherical shape to avoid damage to the blood vessels, and special attention is being given to the distal region of the guidewire to impart to it the appropriate level of flexibility and maneuverability for pVAD implantation. Finally, various hemocompatible coating materials are being tested to provide hemophilic or hemophobic character to the guidewire. For instance, a guidewire coated with silicone is shown in Fig. 5.5c. Numerical simulations using Ansys are in progress to assess various guidewire designs and tests such as the perforation test (to assess the tip shape and its safety), and tests for pushability and trackability are in progress to characterize the fabricated guidewires. For the latter tests, phantoms of the human arterial network are being used, see Fig. 5.6. Such phantoms are 3D printed using suitable materials to replicate the human vasculature in terms of geometry, flexibility, and internal surface texture. Concurrently, catheters consisting of braided tubes embedded inside a flexible material are being designed. A wire braiding machine is being set up and first prototypes are expected to emerge shortly.

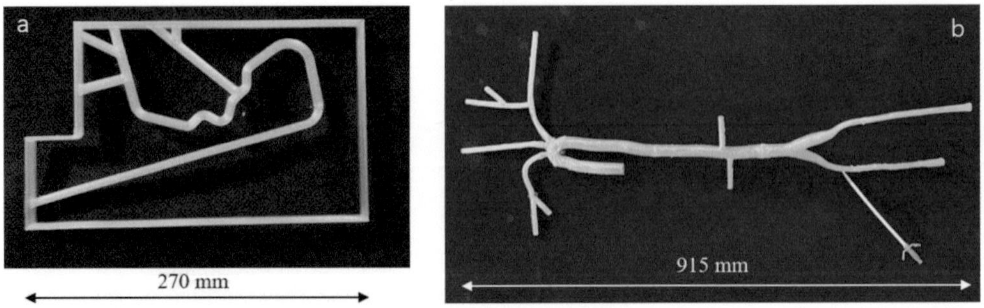


**Fig. 5.6** Phantoms of the vasculature for pushability and trackability tests **a** trackability circuit as per ISO-25539 and **b** phantom of an actual human arterial network

## 5.5 The Path Ahead: Sensors, Device Monitoring, Digital Twins

While considerable progress has been made, several subsystems of the pVAD assembly need to be perfected before various components can be integrated to generate the device prototype. Micromotor, packaged control electronics and user interface, catheters, and a high-performance blood pump are expected to be developed soon. In vitro performance tests of the device with human blood and under dynamic conditions using an advanced test bed will follow. In addition to the above, miniature sensors may be integrated with the device, and their output monitored continuously. Such sensors may be important for the precise positioning of the pVAD across the aortic valve and real-time monitoring of the device's performance. In addition to enhancing treatment outcomes for the patient, such data can also help in further device development. This development may also involve a digital twin, a mathematical/computational model of the device that is continuously fine-tuned based on real-time device data. The model, in turn, can predict the future performance of the device and can advise preemptive interventions in case of anticipated complications.

## 5.6 Outlook: Medical Device Ecosystem

The only pVAD currently available in the country is of a foreign make and is imported. Consequently, its cost is significantly high, prohibiting its wide use. The objective of the current project is two-fold. First, it aims to develop a device that will perform better than the one available in the market and will be priced significantly lower. Second, it will lead to the generation of indigenous capability for the design and manufacture of medical devices. The pVAD comprises several high-end subsystems such as the catheter and guide wire, blood pump, micromotor, and control electronics. Most of these subsystems have a wide range of applications in medical devices. For instance, guidewires and catheters are used in all cathlab procedures, miniaturized high-speed motors can be used, e.g., in dental applications, arterial phantoms for testing biomedical components and training medical staff, and blood pumps in various blood handling devices. Developing these subsystems will not only lead to the development of percutaneous VAD and similar devices but also to an ecosystem for medical device manufacturing in the country.

**Acknowledgements** The article is based on the work done by Pavan Pandit, Ashok Vishwakarma, Jabi Ali, Mohammad Owais, Aditya Rathore, Mandeep Singh Rana, Bhrigu Nath, and Arun Kumar Pandey. We thank IIT Kanpur for funding these activities and Manoj Sharma, Phool Chand Gond, and H.P. Sharma for their support. The team has also received critical input from Dr. Satyendra Tewari and Dr. Shantanu Pande from Sanjay Gandhi Postgraduate Institute of Medical Sciences (SGPGIMS), Lucknow, and Dr. Julius Punnen from Narayana Health, Bangalore.

## References


1. Prabhakaran D, Jeemon P, Roy A (2016) Cardiovascular diseases in India: current epidemiology and future directions. Circulation 133. https://doi.org/10.1161/CIRCULATIONAHA.114.008729
2. Van Edom CJ, Gramegna M, Baldetti L, Beneduce A, Castelein T, Dauwe D, Frederiks P, Giustino G, Jacquemin M, Janssens SP, Panoulas VF, Pöss J, Rosenberg A, Schaubroeck HAI, Schrage B, Tavazzi G, Vanassche T, Vercaemst L, Vlasselaers D, Vranckx P, Belohlavek J, Gorog DA, Huber K, Mebazaa A, Meyns B, Pappalardo F, Scandroglio AM, Stone GW, Westermann D, Chieffo A, Price S, Vandenbriele C (2023) Management of bleeding and hemolysis during percutaneous microaxial flow pump support: a practical approach. JACC Cardiovasc Interv 16(14):1707–1720. https://doi.org/10.1016/j.jcin.2023.05.043
3. Unoki T, Saku K, Kametani M, Konami Y, Taguchi E, Sawamura T, Nakao K, Sakamoto T (2022) Impella motor current amplitude reflects the degree of left ventricular unloading under ECPELLA support a case report. Int Heart J 63. https://doi.org/10.1536/ihj.22-237

# Imaging Through a Single Optical Fibre

6

Shilpi Gupta and Harshawardhan Wanare

**Abstract**

Non-invasive biomedical imaging is a rapidly developing area, and a multitude of efforts in this domain are being pursued worldwide. One of the key challenges is to access hard to reach areas in-vivo with tools that have miniscule footprint and yet provide information with sufficient spatial resolution over a significant imaging volume. We describe here the state-of-the-art and our efforts in this direction.

**Keywords**

Non-invasive imaging · Multimode optical fibre · Speckle · Image reconstruction

## 6.1 Introduction

The ability to image hard-to-reach regions in a minimally invasive manner can be a game changer in the medical domain. The possible use case scenarios range from observing brain activity to disease identification, from tracking the structural to functional aspects of the brain, and in a plethora of endoscopic procedures. All the above scenarios rely on extreme miniaturization of the optical probe, which if realized, promises to be transformative on multiple levels including significantly enhanced patient experience, near negligible damage to the surrounding tissue, and a provision to access the spectral response of the tissue for disease identification in real time. If one has seen or undergone a GI tract endoscopic procedure, one would immediately connect with the patient trauma that it entails, and hence, a reduction in the footprint of the probe would be immensely valuable.

A typical optical fibre has the intrinsic potential to deliver such miniaturization, with a diameter of just 125 μm that is comparable to a human hair, and without significantly compromising the underlying capacity for information transfer as the fibre can support thousands of modes. However, miniaturization imposes a fundamental trade-off between the extent of miniaturization of the optical probe and the performance of the probe. The miniaturized size leads to increased aberration resulting in reduced resolution and a limited field of view. All these challenges need to be addressed simultaneously for deployment of such an imaging tool.

S. Gupta
Department of Electrical Engineering, Indian Institute of Technology Kanpur, Kanpur, India
e-mail: shilpig@iitk.ac.in

H. Wanare (✉)
Department of Physics, Indian Institute of Technology Kanpur, Kanpur, India
e-mail: hwanare@iitk.ac.in

S. Gupta · H. Wanare
Gangwal School of Medical Sciences and Technology, Indian Institute of Technology Kanpur, Kanpur, India


S. Verma (ed.), *Technology and Innovation in Medical Sciences*, IITK Directions 7,
https://doi.org/10.1007/978-981-96-8606-3_6

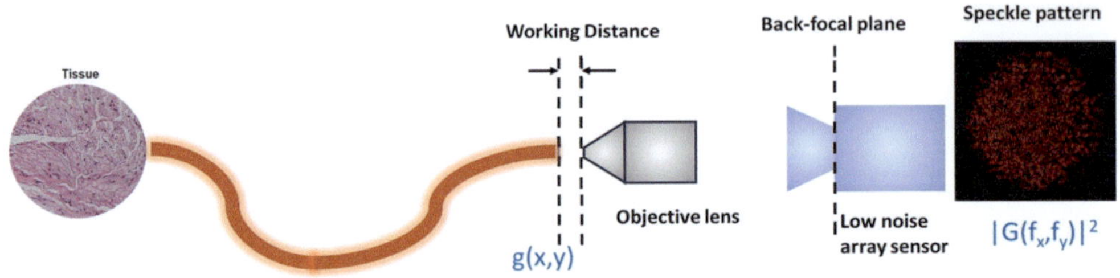


**Fig. 6.1** Schematic of the imaging setup wherein a tissue sample on the left (distal end) when imaged through an optical fibre leads to formation of speckle pattern shown on the right (proximal end) as recorded by the camera

There have a been a variety of developments worldwide in this domain and at the moment we do not have a win-all-solution for the same. We present here the main obstacles and understand the solutions that have been tried across the world, each valuable in a limited setting, and look at the way ahead towards a wholesome solution to this challenging open problem.

## 6.2 Optical Fibre and Associated Challenges

Optical fibres have been central to the information age that we live in. An optical fibre is a narrow flexible glass tube, which guides propagation of light with negligible loss. The cylindrical confinement, accorded by the tube-like geometry of the optical fibre, supports specific spatial solutions of the Maxwell's equations such as the Hermite–Gaussian and Bessel–Gaussian functions that are called the "modes" of the fibre [1].

Optical fibres are categorized based on the refractive index distribution within the cylindrical geometry and the diameter of the fibre. The broad categories include single mode fibres, graded index fibres and multimode fibres. Single mode fibres and graded index fibres allow only one/few modes to propagate in the fibre. These fibres have been used for imaging applications by forming a fibre bundle (comprising of several thousands of single mode fibres) that provides one-to-one mapping of pixelated information between the input and the output ends (one fibre mapping to one pixel on the camera) and thus leading to image formation [2]. A similar approach involves design of a specialty multi-core fibre, again providing a one-to-one mapping from a core to a pixel of the camera [3]. However, both these approaches–one with the fibre bundle and the other with the multicore fibre–have their accompanying limitations such as the overall size of the probe becoming large as the pixel number increases and an uncontrolled coupling between the light modes propagating through the individual cores, respectively [1–3].

In contrast, a multimode fibre (MMF) supports thousands of modes and thus potentially can carry enormous amounts of information–an essential ingredient for imaging [2, 3]. The biggest challenge with a MMF, however, arises from the fact that the light launched into the MMF gets distributed among the multitude of modes within the fibre, suffering from both modal dispersion and intermodal coupling. A typical input–output protocol is shown as a schematic in Fig. 6.1, wherein light scattered from a tissue sample is collected at the input end, which results in random light distribution within the fibre modes, creating a distribution of bright and dark regions known as a speckle pattern at the output end.

Furthermore, any tiny perturbation alters coupling between these modes, and thus, further randomizes the energy distribution within thousands of fibre modes. The random redistribution of energy among the modes in turn alters the spatial pattern of the light at the output end, destroying the object-image mapping essential for imaging. In other words, any slight perturbation to the geometry of the multimode fibre prevents a reliable one-to-one mapping between the spatial location at the input (object) and output (image) ends of the fibre. The perturbations that lead to uncontrolled exchange of energy between modes could arise from a small movement of the fibre, bending of the fibre, twist, or compression of the fibre, as well as scattering within the fibre [4]. This results in dynamic variation of the speckle distribution at the output end. However, the speckle pattern and its correlations have been used to achieve lens-less fibre-bundle imaging in Refs. [5, 6]. The fibre bundle-based and the multicore fibre systems have the potential to offer other multiple advantages, including enabling high resolution histological imaging capable of real-time tumour diagnosis [7]. Even though these technologies are based on fibre bundles, a single MMF can in principle accrue all these capabilities, and thus, offer immense potential.

The major drawbacks associated with the MMF that need to be addressed are the limited field of view, limited ability to offer colour images, and bend sensitivity apart from the intrinsic modal dispersion and intermodal coupling discussed earlier. While these drawbacks have been individually addressed through specialty multicore fibre solutions, for example: Widefield illumination and detection has been extensively investigated using specialty multicore fibres [8]; the limited field of view has also been addressed using coded aperture and a multicore fibre [9], however, the multicore fibres are limited by degradation of image quality due to crosstalk between fibre cores as well as pixelation artefacts [10].

Addressing all these issues can lead to a powerful real-time imaging solution that is compact and low-cost, making it clinically promising for single-use probes as well.

## 6.3 Input–Output Object-Image Mapping Through MMF

In theory, any optical system including a disordered medium like the MMF can be characterized by transmission constants that are complex, implying amplitude and phase information. Such complex valued relationship between the input and output fields (not intensity) is mediated by a complex valued matrix known as the transmission matrix/linear response function/ transfer function. The complex elements of this matrix capture the evolution of the input field amplitude and phase through the disordered medium resulting in the output fields with appropriate phases. Traditionally, the matrix accounts for the fields either in the orthogonal set of modes of the fibre or the spatial frequency modes. The input–output relation is linear, and hence permits, a succinct transfer matrix-based treatment. However, the conventional measurement protocols involve cameras that capture the light intensity (modulus square of light field) and hence the phase information is lost and needs to be additionally captured through an extensive interferometric measurement [11]. An interferometric measurement requires an involved experimental arrangement of an optical reference arm that significantly degrades the system stability. In the context of a single optical probe in an endoscopic arrangement such a referencing for phase retrieval is impractical and would defeat the purpose.

While the relationship between the input intensity and the output intensity of a MMF is not exactly linear, there have been a few efforts towards recasting the relationship through a "pseudo-linear" mapping [12]. The geometry shown in Fig. 6.1 is typical of an endoscopic arrangement wherein limited input-end (object) information needs to be mapped on to the output-end (raw image) that is being accessed by the digital camera that provides a large array of pixels for measurement. Thus, in the pixelated basis the dimensions of the image $I_M$ are $M = p \times q$ and of the object $O_N$ are $N = r \times s$. In practice, the dimensions of the object and the image can be vastly different, and typically $M \gg N$, and thus, rendering the transfer matrix T to be rectangular with real number entries. The resulting transfer matrix connects the output image intensity to the input image intensity in the pixelated basis as following:

$$O_N = T_{N \times M} \cdot I_M$$

An appropriate choice of the basis is critical in determining the transfer matrix in a meaningful manner. Zhao et al. have taken recourse to a shifted set of Hadamard basis [12], that eventually requires a measurement of a combinatorial set of (0, 1) s arranged at the input end with varying periodicities. These periodicities intricately relate diffraction to the pixelated imaging basis. The Hadamard basis offers a full set of input patterns that systematically provides all the requisite set of 2D Fourier modes at the input plane of the optical fibre probe. This exhaustive Fourier mode response allows capturing random input images with sufficient precision. It should be noted that through this intensity-based approach the eventual image needs to be further binarized to obtain the input side intensity pattern of (0, 1 )s. These processes, undertaken in real-time, accomplish the imaging task to a certain extent.

The determination of the transfer matrix is one of the challenges. Additionally, the transfer matrix is extremely sensitive to fibre perturbations including bending, it offers limited field of view, and obtaining the inverse of the transfer matrix is challenging due to lack of mathematical stability–all of these aspects are critical to achieve reliable reconstruction of an image through a single fibre-based endoscope.

## 6.4 Conclusion

Imaging with a single optical fibre is a challenging and an open problem. Incorporating insights from various domains of engineering would allow us to move towards a field deployable single optical fibre imaging tool. The potential for such a device can be a game changer with innumerable applications. Apart from endoscopy, it being used as a surgical lighting aid with an additional functionality of real-time imaging, a viable alternative to peep into a functioning brain, and a host of paediatric use cases. The traditional limitations including resolution, volume-imaging and real-time rendition of images are aspects that continue to be a challenge. We are addressing these challenges by taking recourse to physics guided machine learning tools that can augment the experimental data and realize real time imaging through an MMF.

**Acknowledgements** The generous support from IIT Kanpur under the aegis of the Gangwal School of Medical Sciences and Technology is gratefully acknowledged.

## References

1. Agrawal GP (2010) Fibre-optic communication systems, In: 4th edition (Wiley Series in Microwave and Optical Engineering)
2. Plöschner M, Tyc T, Čižmár T (2015) Seeing through chaos in multimode fibres. Nat Photonics 9(8):529–535
3. Andresen ER, Sivankutty S, Tsvirkun V, Bouwmans G, Rigneault H (2016) Ultrathin endoscopes based on multicore fibres and adaptive optics: a status review and perspectives. J Biomed Opt 21(12):121506
4. Schermer RT, Cole JH (2007) Improved bend loss formula verified for optical fibre by simulation and experiment. IEEE J Quantum Electron 43:899–909
5. Porat A, Andresen ER, Rigneault H et al (2016) Widefield lensless imaging through a fibre bundle via speckle correlations. Opt Express 15:16835–16855
6. Shekel N, Katz O (2020) Using fibre-bending-generated speckles for improved working distance and background rejection in lensless micro-endoscopy. Opt Lett 45:4288–4291
7. Wu J, Wang T, Uckermann O et al (2022) Learned end-to-end high-resolution lens-less fibre imaging towards real-time cancer diagnosis. Sci Rep 12:18846
8. Shahmoon A, Aharon S, Kruchik O, Hohmann M, Solvin H, Douplik A, Zalevsky Z (2013) In vivo minimally invasive interstitial multi-functional microendoscopy. Sci Rep 3:1805
9. Shin J, Tran DN, Stroud JR, Chin S, Tran TD, Foster MA (2019) A minimally invasive lens-free computational microendoscope. Sci Adv 5:eaaw5595
10. Andresen ER, Sivankutty S, Tsvirkun V, Bouwmans G, Rigneault H (2016) Ultrathin endoscopes based on multicore fibres and adaptive optics: a status review and perspectives. J Biomed Opt 21:121506–121506
11. Popoff S, Lerosey G, Carminati R, Fink M, Boccara A, Gigan S (2010) Measuring the transmission matrix in optics: an approach to the study and control of light propagation in disordered media. Phys Rev Lett 104(10):100601
12. Zhao T, Ourselin S, Vercauteren T, Xia W (2020) Seeing through multimode fibres with real-valued intensity transmission matrices. Opt Express 28:20978–20991

# 7 Technological Advancements Transforming Cancer Care: Precision Medicine, AI, and Beyond

Ankita Bhattacharyya, Anjan Roy, and Bushra Ateeq


**Abstract**

Precision medicine has altered the paradigm of cancer research and clinical oncology with improved patient prognosis and outcomes. The advent of high-throughput sequencing technologies and their integration with Machine Learning (ML) and Artificial Intelligence (AI) algorithms have transformed the prospects of cancer care. Moreover, the application of AI/ML models can decode the genomic, epigenomic, and transcriptomic profiles of cancer patients, help in the molecular categorization of cancer patients, and design evidence-based personalized therapeutic strategies. In this article, we discuss some major technological advancements in cancer research, highlighting the role of AI/ML and DL algorithms in the diagnosis and predictive prognosis of cancer patients. We also discuss the utility of liquid biopsy for minimally invasive early cancer detection and treatment. Finally, we highlight the challenges and ethical considerations of AI/ML applications in clinical oncology.



**Keywords**

Precision medicine · Artificial intelligence · Machine learning · Cancer diagnostics · Liquid biopsy · Immuno-oncology


## 7.1 The War Against Cancer—A Quick Recap

Cancer is often described as the 'Emperor of all maladies', referring to a group of diseases where abnormal cells divide uncontrollably, and can spread to distant sites via metastasis [1, 2]. Every year, millions of patients are diagnosed with cancer globally, and more than half of these eventually succumb to death [3, 4]. Despite decades of active research, timely diagnosis and effective treatment of cancer patients remain an unsolved challenge to date.

Historical evidence suggests that the primary treatment of cancer patients involved the surgical removal of tumor tissue aiming at complete disease eradication. However, such intervention proved inefficient for patients with advanced-stage malignancy or upon incomplete removal of tumor mass [5].This was addressed in 1920, when Claudius Renegard discovered the therapeutic potential of using radiation for the treatment of human cancers, with minimal off-target effects. Furthermore, another key turning point in oncology was the advent of chemotherapy in the mid-1900s. Revolutionary findings by Paul Ehrlich demonstrated the use of chemical agents like cytotoxic drugs, alkylating agents, and antimitotic drugs for the treatment of cancer patients, thereby coining the term 'chemotherapy' (Fig. 7.1) [6].


A. Bhattacharyya · A. Roy · B. Ateeq (✉)
Molecular Oncology Laboratory, Department of Biological Sciences and Bioengineering, Indian Institute of Technology Kanpur, Uttar Pradesh, Kanpur, India
e-mail: bushra@iitk.ac.in

B. Ateeq
The Mehta Family Center for Engineering in Medicine, Indian Institute of Technology Kanpur, Uttar Pradesh, Kanpur, India

Centre of Excellence for Cancer, Gangwal School of Medical Sciences and Technology, Indian Institute of Technology Kanpur, Uttar Pradesh, Kanpur, India




S. Verma (ed.), *Technology and Innovation in Medical Sciences*, IITK Directions 7,
https://doi.org/10.1007/978-981-96-8606-3_7

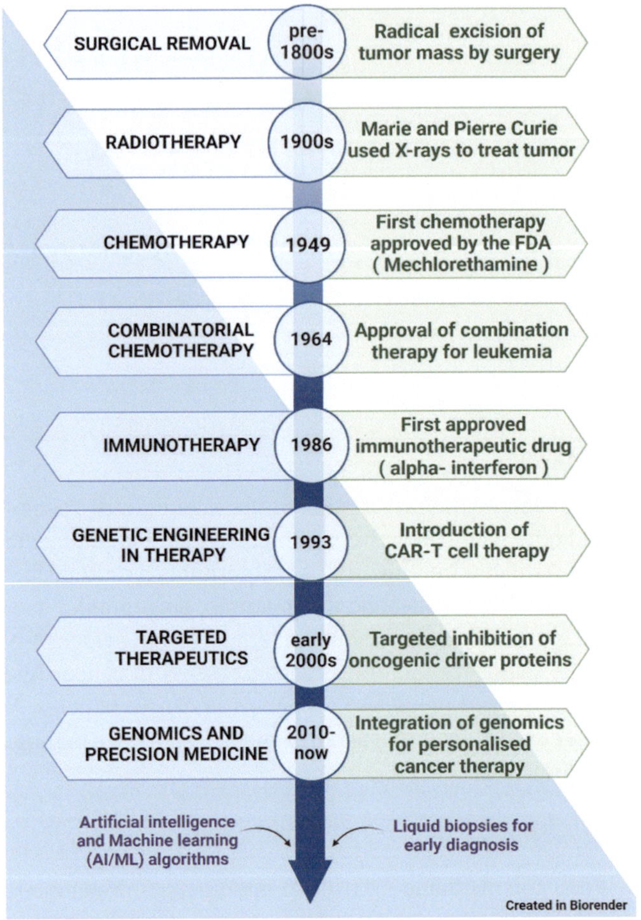


**Fig. 7.1** Milestones in cancer research and therapeutics. Timeline showing the technological advancements in cancer research and integration of AI/ML in cancer therapeutics

While combinatorial treatments using conventional modalities like surgery, chemotherapy, and radiotherapy seemed promising initially, they were also associated with several limitations including lack of specificity and rapid drug metabolism in advanced-stage patients [7]. Dropping this 'one shoe fits all' approach, oncology research introduced the concept of 'precision medicine' and targeted therapeutics. Deviating from the idea of focusing on common factors among patients, precision medicine emphasizes optimizing individualized treatment for higher efficacy [8].

## 7.2 Technological Advancements in Cancer Therapeutics

### 7.2.1 Omics in Precision Oncology

Historical evidence describes three broad eras of medicine—starting with the traditional 'intuition-based medicine', followed by the largely practiced 'evidence-based medicine' with an ongoing shift toward the individualized and personalized approach of 'precision medicine' [9]. In the past few decades, the advent of high-throughput sequencing technologies has revolutionized the field of cancer research and introduced the concept of 'Big data' in oncology, which refers to large, diverse sets of information (genomic data) that are growing at ever-increasing rates. The gradual integration of 'omics' technologies in cancer has generated massive amounts of molecular data requiring extensive infrastructure for its processing and conclusive analysis [10, 11]. The term 'omics' refers to the assimilated characterization and quantification of population datasets, including the genome, transcriptome, proteome, etc. that influence the structural and functional dynamics of a biological process. [9]

A prototypical example of such big data encompasses the information collected as part of the TCGA (The Cancer Genome Atlas), a comprehensive compendium of cancer genome aberrations. This consortium produced genomic, transcriptomic, proteomic and epigenomic data for >20,000 primary cancers and their matched normal specimens spanning 33 different cancers [12]. Integrative analysis of this data unraveled the molecular subtypes of cancers, elucidated their genomic underpinnings, and helped identify therapeutic targets for different tumor types [13]. Other large-scale cancer databases such as the International Cancer Genome Consortium (ICGC), Cancer Cell Line Encyclopedia (CCLE), and the Human Protein Atlas (HPA) have further enriched our understanding of the disease and its pathogenesis [14].

The field of 'Genomics' focuses on decoding the genetic makeup of an individual to unravel the underlying information stored in their DNA (deoxyribonucleic acid) [15]. While they appear to be deceptively simple, the precise arrangement of four nucleotide bases that constitute the DNA double helix forms the crux of the central dogma of molecular biology [16]. Therefore, the accumulation of any abrupt changes in the DNA sequence can alter the function of normal protein, which can lead to the onset and development of cancer [17]. As previously mentioned, such disruptive alterations are studied in large patient cohorts using state-of-the-art next-generation sequencing (NGS) technologies. The Pan-Cancer Atlas generated by the Cancer Genome Atlas (TCGA) network is a prime example of such an initiative [12, 13]. Consequently, the global accessibility of these cancer genomic datasets has further highlighted the molecular heterogeneity and racial disparity across different populations worldwide.

A key advantage of the 'omics' era lies in its precise approach toward the treatment and clinical management of cancer patients. The unified integration of genomic, transcriptomic, and epigenomic datasets of cancer patients brings forth a comprehensive view of patient-specific differences and highlights unique alterations in these individuals. This enables timely diagnosis of the patients, identification of their molecular subtypes, and selection of appropriate therapeutic interventions and better patient outcomes. Although the associated expense for multi-omics data remains a huge challenge, their immense utility in designing customized patient-specific treatments and bypassing therapy resistance makes them an exciting arena for future cancer research and oncology medicine.

### 7.2.2 Pattern Recognition Using AI/ML in Precision Oncology

The past decade has experienced an upsurge in precision oncology with the integration of Big data and AI. Through growing technological advancements, AI and ML algorithms have significantly transformed cancer research in impactful ways [18]. AI/ML applications in oncology include patient risk assessment, timely diagnosis, and predictive patient prognosis based on 'training' data from large-scale cancer datasets [19–21].

In recent times, AI algorithms have been employed for faster processing and more efficient analysis of the extensive data generated from genomic studies, clinical trials, and patient medical records compared to traditional methods. ML is often regarded as the ability of machines to 'think' and includes any computer program that improves its performance at some tasks by 'learning' through experiences [22]. Therefore, ML models can identify distinct patterns and correlations that may not be evident to human researchers, enabling more accurate predictions about cancer risks and outcomes (Fig. 7.2).

Deep Learning (DL) is a crucial subset of AI that has wide-ranging practical utility in oncology healthcare. It is the most frequently used AI tool in cancer diagnostics with diverse applications in medical imaging. DL algorithms allow the interpretation of complex radiological patient data for early detection, characterization, and monitoring of tumor growth and metastases. Furthermore, the inclusion of AI has significantly enhanced the accuracy of the analysis in diagnostic imaging techniques like Magnetic Resonance Imaging (MRI), X-rays, computed tomography (CT/CAT), positron emission tomography (PET), and mammograms [20]. Moreover, AI could be used to predict patient outcomes based on historical data, improve prognosis predictions, and help clinicians make informed decisions about treatment options and follow-up strategies. For example, MammaPrint has currently been used for breast cancer patients with early-stage disease, while a similar method based on a 21-gene signature (Oncotype DX) has been employed to predict the chemotherapy responses in Estrogen Receptor +/–, HER2-negative invasive cases [23, 24].

Despite its suggested potential, the amalgamation of big data and AI/ML with cancer bears its own set of limitations. The high cost, immense computational burden, and associated ethical discrepancies pose a major hurdle to its widespread implementation in global healthcare. Therefore, it is imperative to remove such conundrums, overcome limitations, and adopt the utilization of AI/ML models in routine clinical practices. In summary, the integration of AI in cancer research is enhancing the speed, efficiency, and precision of various aspects of cancer diagnosis and treatment, ultimately leading to improved patient outcomes and a deeper understanding of the disease.

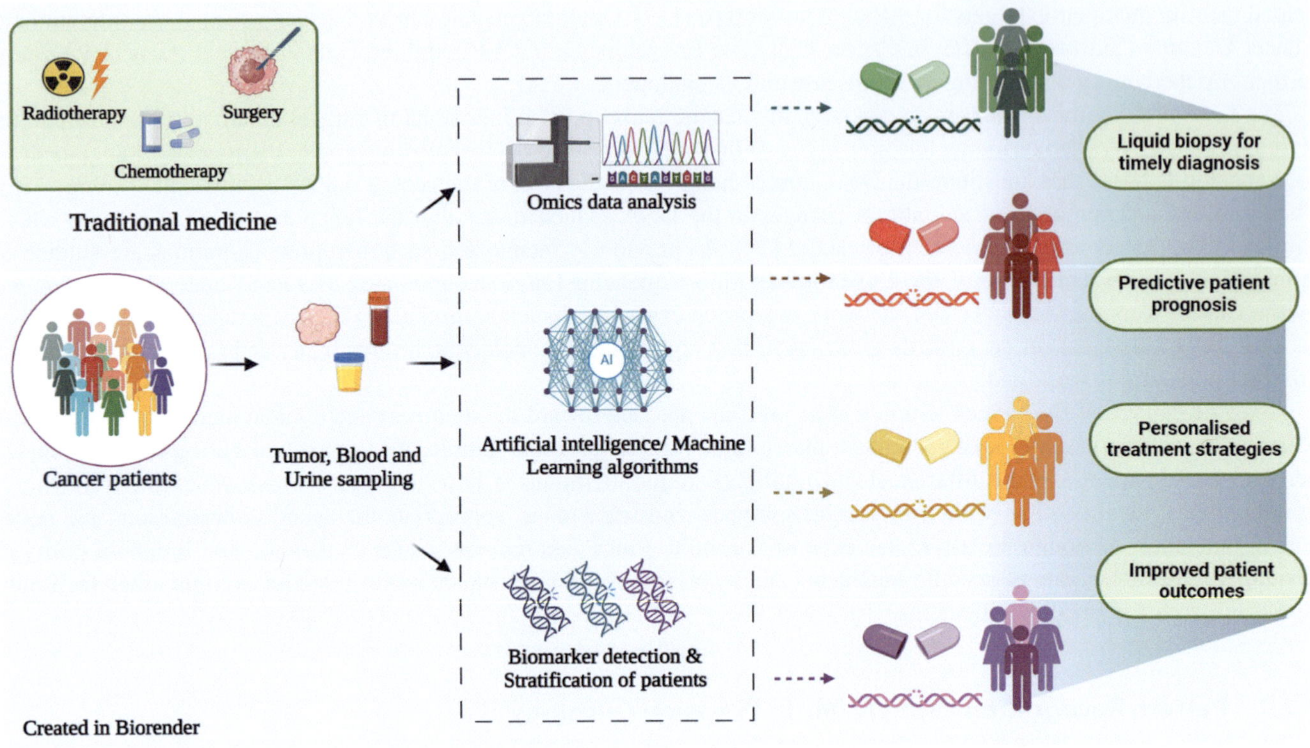


**Fig. 7.2** The paradigm of precision medicine in oncology. Current strategies of precision oncology deviate from the traditional approach involving the integration of chemotherapy, radical surgery, and radiotherapy. Precision medicine involves using patient samples (tumor, blood, or urine) for diagnostic and prognostic purposes. With the rise of AI/ML and DL algorithms, timely diagnosis and personalized treatment strategies help predict patient drug response and ultimately lead to improved patient outcomes

### 7.2.3 Minimally Invasive Cancer Diagnostics

Recent advancements in cancer diagnostics have introduced techniques that avoid tumor tissue sampling and are considered 'minimally invasive'- such as 'liquid biopsy' procedures relying on the patient's body fluids (blood, urine, or other body fluids) to detect biomarkers indicative of cancer. Recent advances have led to the development of liquid biopsies which involve the isolation of tumor-derived entities, such as circulating tumor cells (CTCs), circulating tumor DNA (ctDNA), tumor extracellular vesicles (EVs), etc., present in the body fluids of cancer patients, followed by employing genomics and proteomics characterization methods [25]. Non-invasive methods can provide real-time insight into tumor dynamics and treatment response, facilitating timely adjustments to therapy [22]. For example, circulating nucleic acids encompass ctDNA, which are fragments of tumor DNA representing the genetic and epigenetic repertoire of the main tumor mass. These fragments are usually present at very low concentrations in the patient's blood, thus requiring highly sensitive techniques for their detection [25]. Alternatively, CTCs are cancer cells that sloughed off from the primary tumor and can enter the bloodstream to facilitate distant metastasis. They represent the cellular dynamics of the original tumor tissue, thereby aiding in the early detection of cancers and longitudinal monitoring of patient drug response [26, 27]. Recent studies have also highlighted the utility of EVs in liquid biopsy across multiple cancers. Exosomes are a subtype of EVs that shuttle cellular cargo and mediate intercellular communication. Since cancer-derived exosomes are enriched for tumor-specific surface biomarkers and nucleic acids, they have been demonstrated to be superior to ctDNA and CTCs-based diagnostic methods, which accurately detect cancer and predict patient response [28].

Current strategies opt for a comprehensive approach integrating liquid biopsy with AI/ML strategies for precise diagnosis and patient stratification before treatment. Further, the inclusion of longitudinal studies with genetic and epigenetic data will provide dynamic insights into cancer progression and patient response. A deeper understanding of such molecular events would unravel new therapeutic interventions for cancer patients.

### 7.2.4 Immuno-Oncology in Precision Medicine

An integral part of precision oncology calls for the immune system which should ideally play a central role in eradicating cancer cells from the body. However, cancer cells almost inevitably acquire the ability to 'evade immune destruction', an established hallmark of cancer [29]. A revolutionary keystone in immunotherapeutics was the discovery of the Chimeric Antigen Receptor (CAR) T-cell therapy that utilizes modified immune cells for cancer treatment. Here, the CARs are engineered into T cells that redirect them toward target tumor cells expressing the cognate antigen and precisely eliminate them [30, 31]. These engineered cells also continue to multiply, thereby sustaining a long-term response to act as a living drug [30]. The recent approval of CAR-T cell therapy for the clinical management of patients suffering from liquid malignancy further demonstrates its potential for other cancers [32, 33]. However, this treatment regimen has some major drawbacks including antigen escape, on-target off-tumor effects, and the toxicity associated with CAR-T cell therapy [31].

Another key component of the immune system are the natural killer (NK) cells which also recognize and kill tumor cells [34]. Considering their anti-tumorigenic effect, NK cell therapies have also emerged as a promising strategy for treating cancer patients. Recently, CAR-NK cell therapy was also found to be effective in treating lymphoid cancer patients without any major complications [35]. Other advancements in immunotherapy involve the administration of monoclonal antibodies (mAbs), which recognize target antigens present on cancer cells and selectively eliminate them [36]. Several mAbs have been approved by the Food and Drug Administration (FDA) for the treatment of different malignancies [36].

In the past decade, the integration of genomics data with immunotherapy has led to the advent of personalized vaccines tailored for individual cancer patients. These vaccines are designed after the identification and inhibition of unique/novel targets detected in each patient [37]. A recent study demonstrated the use of personalized neoantigen-targeting vaccines for the treatment of glioblastoma patients [38]. Furthermore, molecular characterization of the immune infiltrates in the surrounding tumor microenvironment has also been established as a key determining factor to improve response rates and develop novel therapeutic interventions for cancer immunotherapy. Considering the complexities associated with tumor–immune microenvironment, technologies such as single-cell sequencing have emerged as powerful tools for deconvoluting molecular heterogeneity of the tumor and its microenvironment.

## 7.3 Conclusion

The comprehensive integration of modern technologies in cancer research has significantly improved patient prognosis and outcomes. While employing AI/ML and DL in cancer care helps increase the efficiency of cancer diagnostics, and reduces chances of human error, strict monitoring should be maintained for ethical concerns including patient privacy, proper medical records, and data security. Therefore, proper ethical guidelines should be enforced to safeguard the consent of the patients, by setting up secure data storage and sharing practices. In addition, another major limitation of the clinical application of advanced minimally invasive diagnostic techniques and immunotherapeutics is the associated high cost and limited affordability. Therefore, current research focuses on reducing treatment costs and enhancing accuracy, and successful clinical translation can significantly improve the therapeutic management of cancer patients in future.

**Acknowledgements** The authors are thankful to the Gangwal School of Medical Sciences and Technology (GSMST) and the Department of Biological Sciences and Bioengineering, Indian Institute of Technology, Kanpur for infrastructural support. The authors thank the India Alliance DBT/Wellcome Trust Senior Fellow (IA/S/19/2/504659), Tata Innovation Fellowship (HRD-16012/6/2024-HRD-DBT), and Department of Biotechnology (DBT/BSBE/2023426) for supporting their research. AB and AR acknowledge the Ministry of Education for the PMRF and CSIR fellowship, respectively. All illustrations in this article were created with BioRender (https://biorender.com/).

## References

1. Hassanpour SH, Dehghani M (2017) Review of cancer from perspective of molecular. J Cancer Res Pract 4:127–129
2. Upadhyay A (2021) Cancer: an unknown territory; rethinking before going ahead. Genes Dis 8:655–661
3. Sung H et al (2021) Global cancer statistics 2020: GLOBOCAN estimates of incidence and mortality worldwide for 36 cancers in 185 countries. CA Cancer J Clin 71:209–249
4. Ferlay J et al (2019) Estimating the global cancer incidence and mortality in 2018: GLOBOCAN sources and methods. Int J Cancer 144:1941–1953

5. Falzone L, Salomone S, Libra M (2018) Evolution of cancer pharmacological treatments at the turn of the third millennium. Front Pharmacol 9
6. DeVita VT, Chu E (2008) A history of cancer chemotherapy. Cancer Res 68:8643–8653
7. Debela DT et al (2021) New approaches and procedures for cancer treatment: current perspectives. SAGE Open Med 9:205031212110343
8. Tsimberidou AM, Fountzilas E, Nikanjam M, Kurzrock R (2020) Review of precision cancer medicine: evolution of the treatment paradigm. Cancer Treat Rev 86:102019
9. Eledkawy A, Hamza T, El-Metwally S (2024) Precision cancer classification using liquid biopsy and advanced machine learning techniques. Sci Rep 14:5841
10. Dai X, Shen L (2022) Advances and trends in omics technology development. Front Med (Lausanne) 9
11. Jiang P et al (2022) Big data in basic and translational cancer research. Nat Rev Cancer 22:625–639
12. Weinstein JN et al (2013) The cancer genome atlas pan-cancer analysis project. Nat Genet 45:1113–1120
13. Hutter C, Zenklusen JC (2018) The cancer genome atlas: creating lasting value beyond its data. Cell 173:283–285
14. Wu X, Li W, Tu H (2024) Big data and artificial intelligence in cancer research. Trends Cancer 10:147–160
15. Minchin S, Lodge J (2019) Understanding biochemistry: structure and function of nucleic acids. Essays Biochem 63:433–456
16. Crick F (1970) Central dogma of molecular biology. Nature 227:561–563
17. Stratton MR, Campbell PJ, Futreal PA (2009) The cancer genome. Nature 458:719–724 Preprint at https://doi.org/10.1038/nature07943
18. Patnaik D, Patnaik S (2024) New paradigm in financial technology using machine learning techniques and their applications, pp 467–483. https://doi.org/10.1007/978-3-031-61037-0_22
19. Iqbal MJ et al (2021) Clinical applications of artificial intelligence and machine learning in cancer diagnosis: looking into the future. Cancer Cell Int 21:270
20. Dlamini Z, Francies FZ, Hull R, Marima R (2020) Artificial intelligence (AI) and big data in cancer and precision oncology. Comput Struct Biotechnol J 18:2300–2311
21. Zhang B, Shi H, Wang H (2023) Machine learning and AI in cancer prognosis, prediction, and treatment selection: a critical approach. J Multidiscip Healthc 16:1779–1791
22. Pammi M, Aghaeepour N, Neu J (2023) Multiomics, artificial intelligence, and precision medicine in perinatology. Pediatr Res 93:308–315
23. Kaklamani V (2006) A genetic signature can predict prognosis and response to therapy in breast cancer: oncotype DX. Expert Rev Mol Diagn 6:803–809
24. Rafique R, Islam SMR, Kazi JU (2021) Machine learning in the prediction of cancer therapy. Comput Struct Biotechnol J 19:4003–4017
25. Foser S, Maiese K, Digumarthy SR, Puig-Butille JA, Rebhan C (2024) Looking to the future of early detection in cancer: liquid biopsies, imaging, and artificial intelligence. Clin Chem 70:27–32
26. Lawrence R, Watters M, Davies CR, Pantel K, Lu Y-J (2023) Circulating tumour cells for early detection of clinically relevant cancer. Nat Rev Clin Oncol 20:487–500
27. Deng Z, Wu S, Wang Y, Shi D (2022) Circulating tumor cell isolation for cancer diagnosis and prognosis. EBioMedicine 83:104237
28. Yu D et al (2022) Exosomes as a new frontier of cancer liquid biopsy. Mol Cancer 21:56
29. Hanahan D (2022) Hallmarks of cancer: new dimensions. Cancer Discov 12:31–46 Preprint at https://doi.org/10.1158/2159-8290.CD-21-1059
30. Sadelain M, Brentjens R, Rivière I (2013) The basic principles of chimeric antigen receptor design. Cancer Discov 3:388–398 Preprint at https://doi.org/10.1158/2159-8290.CD-12-0548
31. Sterner RC, Sterner RM (2021) CAR-T cell therapy: current limitations and potential strategies. Blood Cancer J 11 Preprint at https://doi.org/10.1038/s41408-021-00459-7
32. Kochenderfer JN et al (2010) Eradication of B-lineage cells and regression of lymphoma in a patient treated with autologous T cells genetically engineered to recognize CD19. Blood 116:4099–4102
33. Grupp SA et al (2013) Chimeric antigen receptor-modified T cells for acute lymphoid leukemia. N Engl J Med 368:1509–1518
34. Malmberg KJ et al (2017) Natural killer cell-mediated immuno surveillance of human cancer. Semin Immunol 31:20–29 Preprint at https://doi.org/10.1016/j.smim.2017.08.002
35. Liu E et al (2020) Use of CAR-transduced natural killer cells in CD19-positive lymphoid tumors. N Engl J Med 382:545–553
36. Zahavi D, Weiner L (2020) Monoclonal antibodies in cancer therapy. Antibodies 9:1–20 Preprint at https://doi.org/10.3390/antib9030034
37. Blass E, Ott PA (2021) Advances in the development of personalized neoantigen-based therapeutic cancer vaccines. Nat Rev Clin Oncol 18:215–229 Preprint at https://doi.org/10.1038/s41571-020-00460-2
38. Keskin DB et al (2019) Neoantigen vaccine generates intratumoral T cell responses in phase Ib glioblastoma trial. Nature 565:234–239

# Collaborative Robots in Operative Dentistry 8

Abhinav sharma, Rahul Sagwal, Deepak Mishra,
and J. Ramkumar

**Abstract**

Dentistry is an expanding market and a challenging profession that deals with a broad spectrum of oral health issues. It is characterized by complex procedural guidelines and an extremely high patient-to-dentist ratio resulting in heavy workloads and stress for professionals. Furthermore, a significant number of dental offices carry out their activities in work areas that are not ergonomically optimized which means occupational risks are present, i.e., musculoskeletal disorders. This paper describes the current problems in contemporary dentistry and discusses the possibilities of technological approaches. A case study is provided in order to illustrate the use of collaborative robots (cobots) to address these issues. The combination of innovative robotics such as cobots and exoskeleton devices is a potential avenue for enhancing dental practice. In addition, progress in medical imaging, and artificial intelligence (AI), is on the cusp of transforming the diagnostic process and treatment pathways and providing increased accuracy and efficiency. The combination of robot, AI, and imaging technologies, not only simplifies workflow process, but also enhances the quality of services and treatment for patients. With the development of the field, implementation of such innovation will prove to be of critical importance in relieving practitioners' fatigue, improving patient satisfactions, and responding to the increasing needs in the field of oral healthcare.

**Keywords**

Dentistry · Collaborative robots (Cobots) · Medical Technology (Medtech) · Artificial Intelligence (AI)

## 8.1 Introduction

Dentistry is one of the oldest fields of contemporary medicine, its mentions are found in ancient writings. It is an area of concentration on the examination, diagnosis and treatment of oral conditions such as disorders and diseases of the teeth, gums and associated structures. Dental practice involves a broad set of procedures, from basic preventive care to high tech procedures like root canal therapy, extraction and restorations. Dentistry in current times has grown into a multidisciplinary specialty which cares for the wellbeing of the oral cavity in its entirety.

A. sharma · R. Sagwal · D. Mishra · J. Ramkumar (✉)
Department of Design, IIT Kanpur, Kanpur, India
e-mail: jrkumar@iitk.ac.in

A. sharma
e-mail: abhinavs22@iitk.ac.in

R. Sagwal
e-mail: rahuls22@iitk.ac.in

D. Mishra
e-mail: deepakm23@iitk.ac.in


S. Verma (ed.), *Technology and Innovation in Medical Sciences*, IITK Directions 7,
https://doi.org/10.1007/978-981-96-8606-3_8

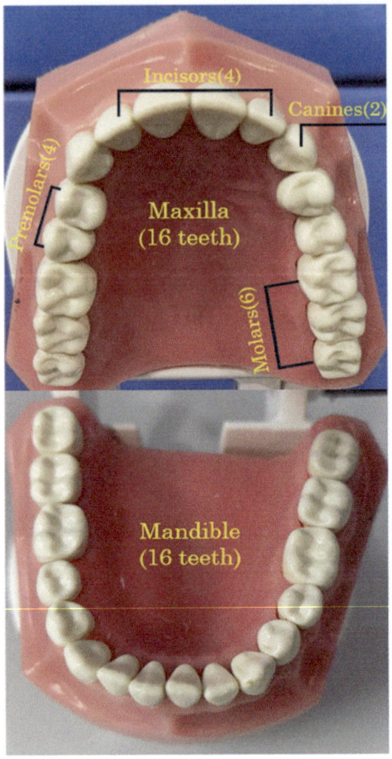


**Fig. 8.1** Dental arcade

## 8.2 Basic Terminology of Dental Arcade

The term dental arcade is the anatomic disposition of the teeth in the mouth, i.e., the curved area of teeth formed by the series of teeth of crowns in the upper and lower jaws. It is commonly employed to characterize the overall form, positioning and structure of teeth in relation to the jaw [1]. Figure 8.1 shows schematic of dental arcade.

1. **Maxillary Arcade**: The dental arcade of the **upper jaw**.
2. **Mandibular Arcade**: The dental arcade of the **lower jaw**.
3. **Arch**: Refers to the shape or curve formed by the dental arcade, resembling a "U" or "V" shape.
4. **Occlusion**: The way the teeth of the upper and lower dental arcades come together when the mouth is closed.
5. **Anterior Teeth**: The teeth located in the front of the dental arcade, including the incisors and canines.
6. **Posterior Teeth**: The teeth located in the back, including premolars and molars.
7. **Diastema**: A gap or space between teeth within the dental arcade.
8. Tooth position and/or alignment on the dental arcade is of a significant importance for chewing, speech, and oral hygiene [2].

## 8.3 Evolution of Dentistry

Dentistry has undergone substantial evolution over the centuries. The oldest evidence of dental treatment comes from ancient Egypt and Mesopotamian civilizations in which crude instruments were employed for tooth extraction and oral hygiene. During the Middle Ages, barber-surgeons performed most of the dental work, mainly extractions. Modern dental practice dates back to eighteenth and nineteenth centuries, with new knowledge in the fields of dental science, analgesia, and hygiene contributing to development of better techniques for tooth restoration and tooth preservation. Pierre Fauchard, the "Father of Modern Dentistry", established methods upon which modern practice is based, for example, fillings and prostheses [3].

In the twentieth century, dentistry experienced rapid growth with the development of X-rays, fluoride treatments, and modern anesthetics, significantly improving diagnosis and treatment. Down through the years, innovations that include digital

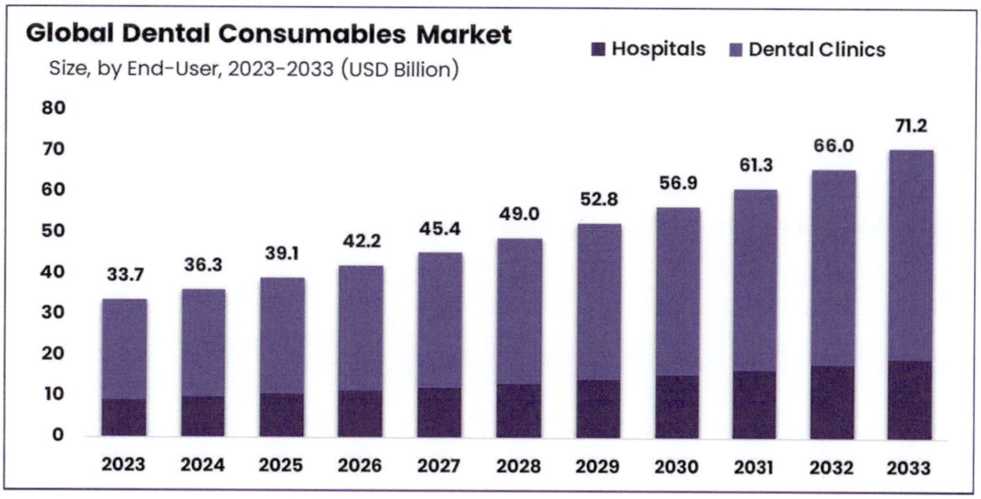


**Fig. 8.2** Global dental market [4]

imaging, laser technology, and computer-aided design and manufacturing (CAD/CAM) have continued to change this field in a more positive and accurate direction while promoting patient comfort.

## 8.4 Market Size of Dentistry

The global dental sector is a big and expanding area of healthcare. In 2023, the global dental market was valued at $33.7 billion and it is projected to reach $56.9 billion in 2030 with a rate of compound annual growth (CAGR) of 7.8% as illustrated by Fig. 8.2 [4]. This expansion is the result of several factors, including increased awareness of oral health, growing popularity for cosmetic dentistry, aging population, and dental technology advancements. Markets in developing countries, particularly in the Asia–Pacific and Latin America, are also rapidly expanding with the rise of good health facilities and increasing purchasing power.

Some of the most important sectors of the dental market are dental services (which are preventive, restorative and surgical treatments), dental products (implant, crown and braces), and dental equipment (e.g., X-ray equipment, dental lasers and CAD/CAM systems.

## 8.5 Technological Challenges in Dentistry

Although there have been great advances in medical technology, dental practice still faces a number of roadblocks in implementation of these novel technologies [5].

- **Cost of Implementation**: Lack of accessibility to high-performance dental technologies, which include 3D imaging systems, lasers and mechanical robotic-assisted tools, due to their high price tag, restricts the general use, especially by small practices and in developing countries.
- **Learning Curve**: In most of the cases, long training represents one of the requirements of the dental professionals who are going to learn and use a new technology, e.g., CAD/CAM systems and digital workflow tools. This slows down their implementation in clinical settings.
- **Regulatory Approvals**: Clinical trials with a high level of rigor and regulatory reviews are necessary to validate the safety and effectiveness of new dental technologies. The approval process is a long and cumbersome one, which will increase time to market entry.
- **Integration with Existing Systems**: Introducing new technologies into established systems, particularly for patient management software and electronic health record, it is a logistical and technological challenge for dental practices.

- **Patient Trust and Acceptance**: There could be some reluctance of patients toward technology-driven procedures, especially if robots or artificial intelligence tools are employed. To ensure the large scale acceptance of these technologies, patients must be informed about the benefits they provide [6].

## 8.6 Scope of Collaborative Robots (Cobots) in Dentistry

Collaborative robots, or "cobots," a type of robot to be operated and utilized for collaborative working with specialized human partners in shared areas, will provide improved accuracy, reduced fatigue and improved efficacy [7]. In dentistry, cobots are capable of changing clinical work flows and patient outcomes, in many ways:

- **Precision in Procedures**: Cobots may be used by the dentists to perform fine tasks requiring precision, such as the preparation of cavities, implant and endodontic treatment. Their capacity to repeat processes with minimal errors can be applied to assist and reduce human error.
- **Reduced Operator Fatigue**: Musculoskeletal disorders and cognitive fatigue may arise from performing repetitive and physically laborious work carried out by dental technicians. Cobots are capable of small repeatable tasks, freeing the dentist's time so that the greater number decision making and treatment planning may still need to be addressed.
- **Improved Patient Safety and Outcomes**: Combining AI and ML algorithms in COBOTs is capable of performing real-time data analysis in conjunction with the execution of a procedure, yielding additional decision support to enhance the patient quality of care by minimizing complications or procedural errors.
- **Automation of Routine Tasks**: Cobots may be used for non-invasive tasks, e.g., the decontamination of instruments, the preparation of materials or the operation of instruments, which can increase the efficiency of the workflow in busy dental practices (e.g., by making a complex task controllable through a single operator).
- **Teaching and Training**: In combination with collaborative robots, such robots can also be applied as training tools in dental education for new dentists. With them it is possible to provide realistic representations of involved processes with students which enable a high level of reproducibility without risk of patient injury.
- **AI Integration**: With the increase in the development of AI-based technologies, cobots are going to be able more and more to learn from past cases, becoming more accurate and allowing dentists to make increasingly correct diagnoses and treatments.

The integration of collaborative robots in dentistry is at the cutting edge of automation and digitization of medicine. Through human dentist skill augmentation cobots, it is possible to enhance the accuracy, speed, and safety of dental procedures. As the dental market gets bigger on a global basis, there is likely to be an increased demand for technology-enabled, higher intensified solutions, which cobots are poised to play an integral role in the next generation of dentistry. However, the problems of cost, training and patient tolerability, will be of significance in the effective use of [8].

## 8.7 The Role of MedTech Labs in Overcoming Challenges and Incorporating Collaborative Robots in Dentistry

Medical technology (Medtech) labs play a critical role for addressing the application of collaborative robots (cobots) in dentistry [9]. These labs are centers of innovation with the function of research, development, and implementation of new technology in medicine. In dentistry, MedTech labs are central to breaking down the technical, organizational and academic barriers to the use of cobots in the clinical setting. The following aspects emphasize the critical functions of MedTech labs in solving problems and speeding up the implementation of collaborative robots in dentistry.

1. **Research and Development of Specialized Robotic Systems**
   MedTech labs are at the forefront of the design and testing of robotic systems to be incorporated under dental conditions. Precision and flexibility are qualities that demand by Dentistry and traditional robotic systems may not be out of the box [10]. MedTech laboratories counter this by creating the hardware and software components necessary for a dental procedure in isolation. These labs create cobots that can carry out complex tasks, such as drilling or treating teeth, alongside dental practitioners. Innovations include:

   a. **Advanced Sensors**: MedTech laboratories are designing sensitive interface between high performance sensors and cobots to ensure real-time control and accuracy of during an operation, i.e., implant insertion, or cavity preparation. These sensors enable the cobots to provide fine haptic feedback to clinicians performing even complex procedures, such as dentists.
   b. **Machine Learning and AI**: Research in the MedTech labs centers around the integration between artificial intelligence (AI) and cobots. Using machine learning, these cobots can be adapted to the patient anatomy and learn from similar procedures, in return increasing accuracy and decreasing errors on the fly.
2. **Prototyping and Testing**
   One of the biggest issues with implementing CRP in dentistry is in safety, reliability and practicality in the clinic. MedTech labs make prototypes and go through a large amount of bench testing as part of the refinement of cobot designs prior to their clinical deployment in dental offices. The iterative cycle of testing and redesigning robotic systems enables MedTech investigators to tackle critical issues related to safety mechanisms, ergonomic designs, and user interfaces.
   a. **Simulation and Testing Models**: MedTech laboratory applies 3D modeling, virtual reality (VR) and simulation techniques for evaluating performance of the cobots in virtual environments prior to clinical trials. This method enables the identification and resolution of clinically safe technical problems.
   b. **Collaboration with Dental Experts**: MedTech labs in collaboration with teeth wearers (dentists, dental educators, and other health care professionals) collaboratively conduct cobot usability tests in a real world setting. Feedback from these practitioners is used to evolve the design of the cobots for easy and practical use, such as in the routine dental practice setting.
3. **Cost Reduction Through Technological Innovation**
   Acquisition and implementation of cobots is one of the main challenges in implementing cobots in the dentistry. MedTech labs are researching and developing ways to reduce cobot system costs by looking at alternative materials, production methods, and economies of scale in fabrication.
   a. **Optimizing Robotic Design**: Modular designs are used to offer tool manufacturers ways to make builds and cobots that can be specified on the needs of individual dental practices. This, consequently, makes it less necessary for costly, specialized systems, and makes cobots feasible in smaller clinics.
   b. **Open-source Development**: Some MedTech labs focus on open-source software and hardware, such that robotic technology can be used in dental offices at a low cost of expensive proprietary programs (a cheap first generation robot). Open source cobots can make more affordable and individualizable tools available to dental professionals.
4. **Addressing the Learning Curve and Training**
   One major challenge is the steep learning curve that dental clinicians adapted to new technologies such as cobots. MedTech labs are used to enable this in the development of an integrated suite of training and educational materials which ensure dental workers are properly equipped to use collaborative robots.
   a. **Simulation-based Training**: In MedTech labs, the application of advanced simulation facilities allows dentists to "practice on" cobots in a safe environment. These simulations are analogous to dental treatment in the real world, in that dentists can practice on simulation cases without the ethical commitment to treat real patients.
   b. **Collaborative Training Programs**: At MedTech labs, as well as coordinated courses, workshops and certification, are also working with dental schools, universities and professional bodies in order to train dentists and dental assistants in the use of cobots. These pedagogical programs go beyond training in the technical aspects of cobot operation, and their aim is to be incorporated into workflow tasks in dental environments.
   c. **Continuous Learning**: In collaboration with AI developers, MedTech labs are working to create cobots with learning capabilities that assist dentists during live procedures. Once dentists work with these robots, cobots offer real-time feedback and recommendations, which are based on pattern learning from past clinical cases, to enable the "on-the-job" learning.
5. **Regulatory Compliance and Safety Standards**
   Safety and regulatory compliance for collaborative robots in dentistry is an essential step leading to their general application. MedTech labs are essential for performing the required research and trials to comply with the demanding regulatory standards of health authorities and standards organizations.
   a. **Clinical Trials and Data Analysis**: MedTech laboratories are required to design clinical trials to determine the effectiveness and safety of cobots in dentistry. During this trials of data that is deemed important enough to receive approval from agencies such as the ones in the United States, Food and Drug Administration (FDA), European Medicines Agency (EMA) and others, regulatory governmental authorities.

b. **Risk Assessment**: Safety regarding working with collaborative robots should not be underestimated and even less so for the complex task of dentistry. MedTech labs provide tools to design and experiment with failsafe solutions preventing malfunction or accident. In particular, force-limiting capabilities are integrated into cobots for use in dental applications, such that they cease operating if they are either surprised by an unexpected amount of force or an obstruction, thereby safeguarding the patient.

6. **Promoting Patient Acceptance**
Utilization of cobots in dental procedures also depends on patient confidence and acceptance. MedTech laboratories are involved in public education programs aimed at improving understanding of what cobots can do and how to address any anxieties that may be present in relation to robot-assisted dentistry.
   a. **Educational Campaigns**: MedTech labs collaborate with marketers and communicators to create patient-centered materials that explain chatbot operation and what it delivers (e.g., enhanced accuracy, enhanced safety).
   b. **Patient Involvement in Desig**n: In a number of labs, patients participate in the testing phase, letting them see cobot-assisted procedures from the perspective of a user and provide feedback. This can be used to improve the user experience and the user trust toward robotic technology.

MedTech labs play an important role in encouraging the use of collaborative robots in dentistry through the technical, financial, and curricular barriers that accompany these technologies. (MedTech) laboratories are able to aid in the introduction of cobots into the everyday treatment setting by making advanced robotic systems available, lowering the costs, ensuring that these systems meet regulatory requirements, and offering their full range of training capabilities. Moreover, by education of patients and their clinicians, they engender trust in such technologies, and thereby, allow collaborative robots to become an integral part of the dentistry of tomorrow.

## 8.8 Case Study of Application of Cobots in Dentistry [Developed at Medtech Lab, IIT Kanpur]

### 8.8.1 A 3-DOF Collaborative Robot for Periodontal Procedures: An Application Note

Collaborative Robots (COBOTS) have interestingly become part of manufacturing industry given their precision and repeatability in doing a task. In medical applications use of COBOTS is still limited and explored.

In this section, we shall discuss the design of COBOT assisted manual scaling procedure practiced extensively in periodontal clinics. Manual scaling is a tedious and repeated procedure which requires meticulous efforts from the clinician.

The proposed system consists of a 3-DoF manipulator arm with a memory unit to retain the joint positions detected by sensory information. In a typical teach exercise the clinician can move the arm over the parts of teeth subject to investigation. The memory unit retains the joint positions and is capable to repeat the trajectory over specified number of cycles.

The end effectors in the arm are customizable depending on the kind of application practiced by the clinician. In our experiment we have used a manual scaler for cleaning the anterior teeth. The tool is integrated with the arm and redesigned for cohesive motion. A detailed descriptive schematic of the proposed system is shown in Fig. 8.3.

Manipulation of robotic joints controlled virtually or teleoperated are very common but becomes atypical for an environment mutually shared by the human and arm as in our case. To facilitate this a (computer vision-based) Coordinate mapping system is proposed to actively monitor the human activities (both the clinician and the patient) and modify the guided trajectory.

### 8.8.2 Oral Geometry and Coordinate Mapping

The robotic system consists of three distinct units namely the Robotic arm, Flexible Intraoral Scanner and the human patient. To perform the kinematic modeling it becomes essential to align the three different coordinates system. Two popular choices for fixing the reference point origin can be the center of the mouth and the tip of the end effector tool. Although oral cavity center is a natural origin for moving the tool in and out with positive and negative motions but the chances of human head movement are almost certain which changes the entire geometry. To prevent this, we fix the origin to the tool tip at the end effector. To map the coordinate system effectively each joint is assigned a frame of reference in Cartesian system and modeled with respect to a global frame of reference attached to the geometric center of the human mouth. The joint 0 (J1) of the cobot is assigned as its origin for individually controlling the joint positions (Fig. 8.4).

Additional frame of reference is attached to the camera used for monitoring the work space anomaly. To mitigate ambiguity in following the trajectory with precision the tool tip instead of the robot end effector slot is assigned as the final frame of reference and the first joint J1 is assigned as the base frame.

Geometric Modulations in the 3-d movement of the flexible intra oral scanner are mapped to maxima and minima boundary conditions based on the available epidemiological data. Figure 8.5 explains the trigonometric model.

Assuming B to be the farthest point of access (maxima boundary) and A to be the nearest tip to the rigid part of the scan tool we calculate the effective length of motion ($\alpha$) for the flexible part by the Eq. 8.1 given below:

$$\alpha = \sqrt{(y-h)^2 + (x-a)^2} \tag{8.1}$$

Based on this calculations and design constraints we propose here the design of the flexible part of the oral scan tool as shown in Fig. 8.6a and b

The rigid portion of the tool is mounted and supported on the COBOT end effector for driving the roll motion.

Yaw and Pitch motion inside the oral cavity is derived through a compliant mechanism. The mechanism is driven by frictional strings and controlled by servo mechanism. Camera is mounted at the tip of the tool.

The developed system is shown below in Fig. 8.7a and b.

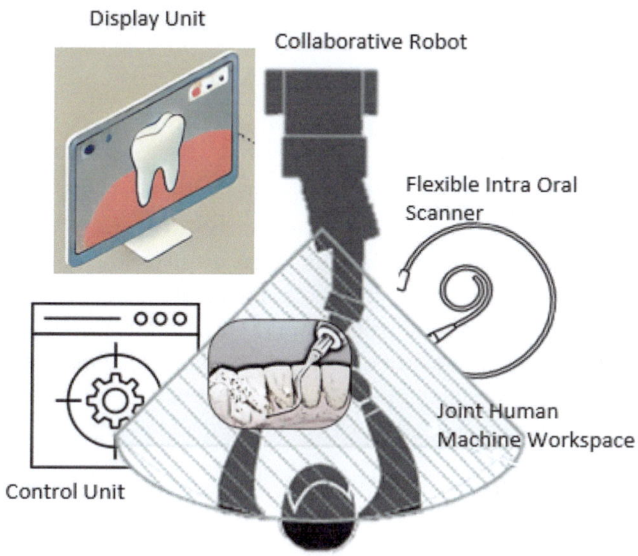


**Fig. 8.3** Schematic diagram of the proposed scaling procedure assisted by a 3-DoF COBOT

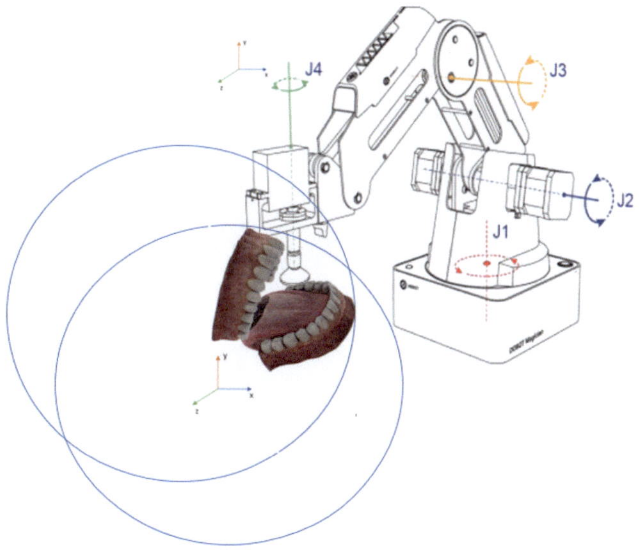


**Fig. 8.4** Spherical co-space and coordinate system for motion planning

With the advent of AI enabled technologies medical practitioners are able to get a more detailed perspective of the treatment. Better visualizations, focused analysis and targeted predictions are helping them in making better healthcare environments. In the next section we shall discuss the potential uses of AI and Machine Learning in dental treatments.

## 8.9 Leveraging AI in Dentistry: Transforming Oral Healthcare in the New Normal Era

### 8.9.1 Role of AI in Modern Dentistry

Artificial Intelligence (AI) and Machine Learning (ML) in modern dentistry are predominantly applied to augment human decision-making by processing vast amounts of medical data. With AI's capabilities in data & image processing, pattern recognition, text generation, predictive analysis, and resource's optimization, dentistry has witnessed tremendous advancements in disease early detection, diagnostics, treatment planning, material optimal utilization, enhanced patient care & experience, and overall workflow improvement [11]. Additionally, cutting edge AI & optimization technologies enhance clinical decision making, operational efficiency, and treatment personalization. Machine Learning based models outstand traditional practices when it comes to recognizing patterns in dental radiographs, image-based diagnostics, 3D cone-beam computed tomography (CBCT) scans, and intraoral images that might not be clearly visible to the naked human eyes. This part further elucidates branches of dentistry, intricacies of dental imaging, application of AI tools in these branches and the challenges associated with it. Refer Fig. 8.8 for word cloud representation of terminologies used in dentistry and AI.

## 8.10 Branches of Dentistry and Application of AI

Figures 8.9 and 8.10 elucidate the different branches of dentistry and application of AI in them.

Graphical Literature Survey of branches of dentistry while integrating AI in operational practices as represented in Fig. 8.11

In addition to CNNs there are many more machine learning techniques that find application in prediction tasks, personalization of scheduling & treatment, image processing for early detection of oral cancer and other diseases, dentistry robotics and analysis of patient behaviors [13]. These ML techniques and their applications are shown, refer Fig. 8.12.

The synergy between robotics, AI, and imaging technologies not only streamlines workflows but also improves the quality of care delivered to patients. As the field evolves, adopting these innovations will play a pivotal role in reducing practitioner fatigue, enhancing patient outcomes, and addressing the growing demands of oral healthcare.

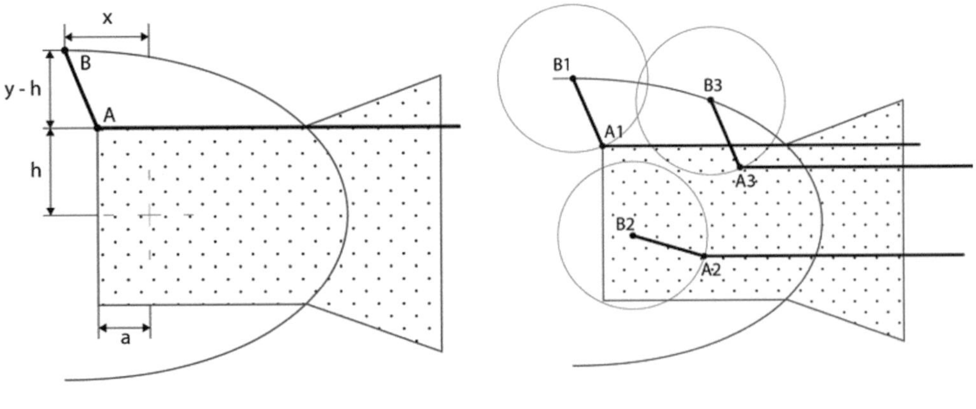


**Fig. 8.5** Trigonometric model of the oral cavity

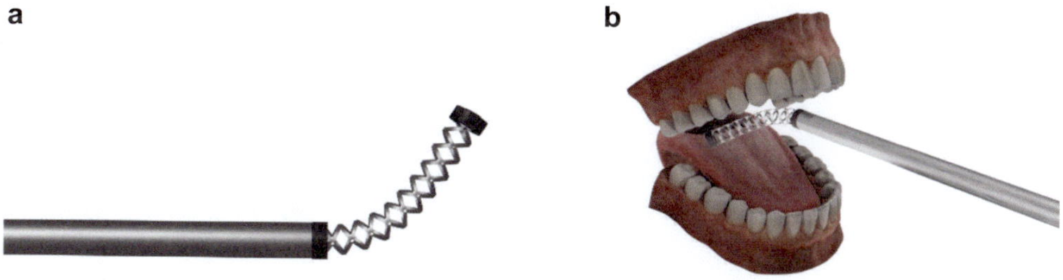

**Fig. 8.6** **a** Flexible intra oral scan tool, **b** Mount of the scan tool in the oral cavity

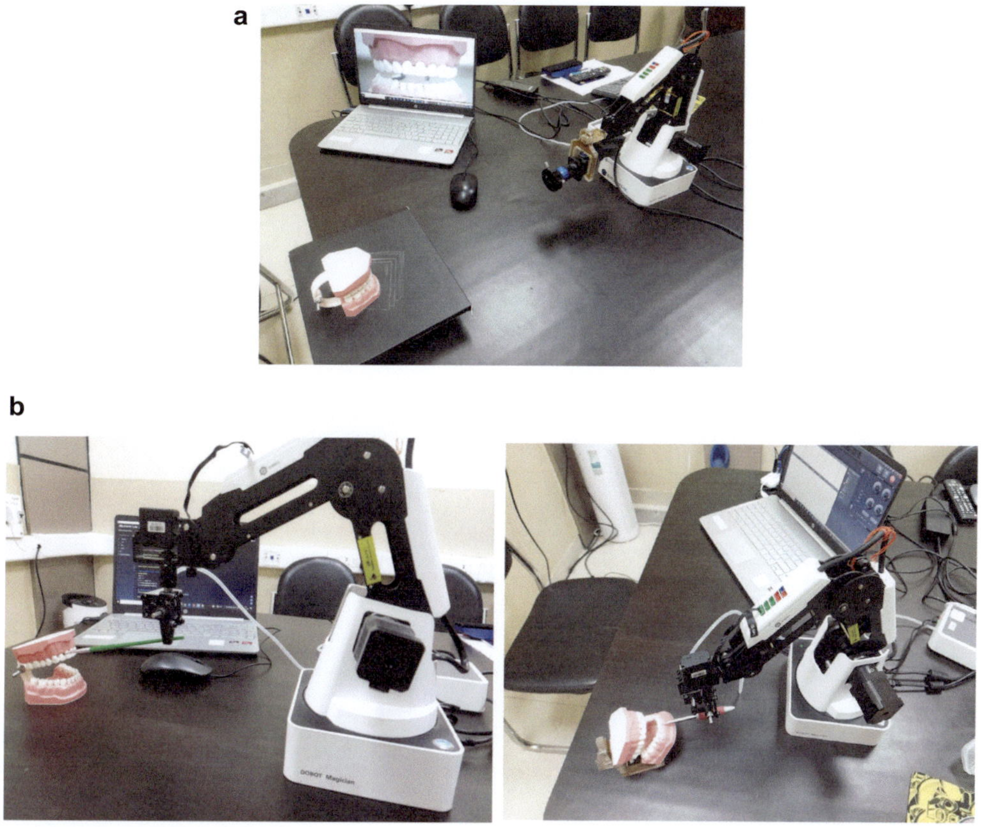

**Fig. 8.7** **a** COBOT and stereo vision system, **b** Cleaning and Scaling operation on dental arch using COBOT

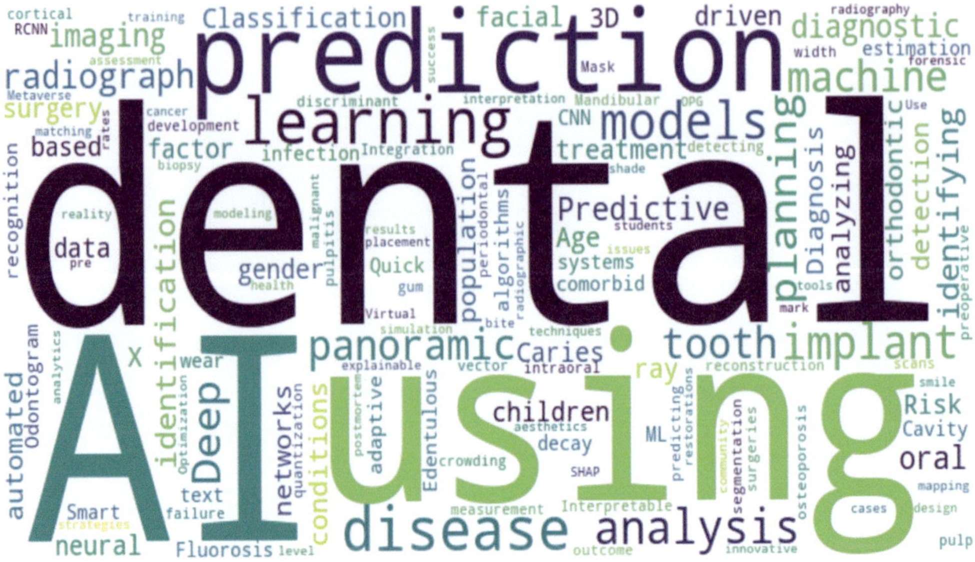


**Fig. 8.8** Word cloud representation of AI and dental terminologies

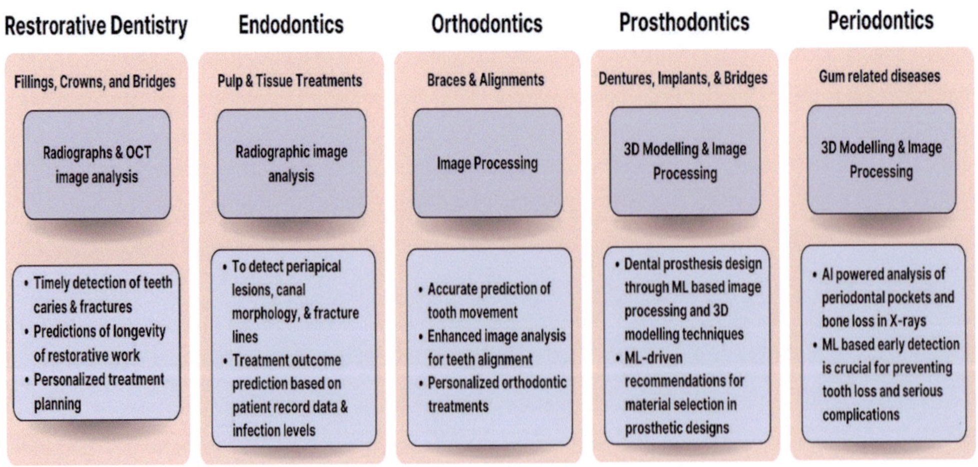


**Fig. 8.9** Summary of use of AI in operative dentistry

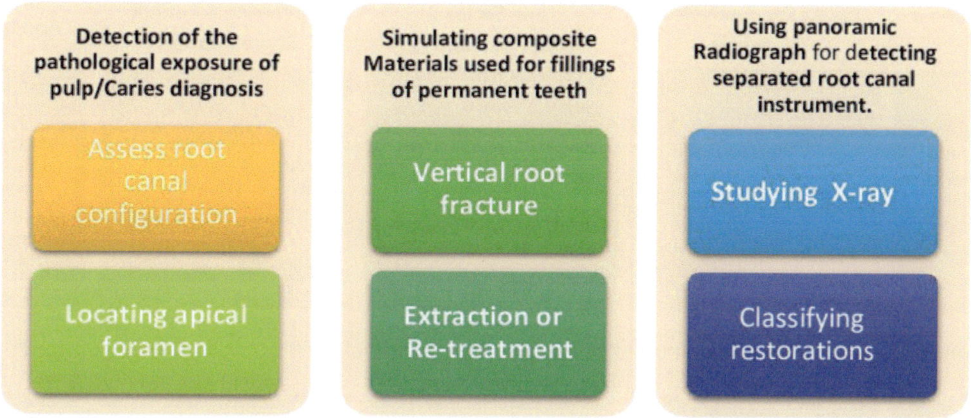


**Fig. 8.10** Summary of use of AI in endodontics [12]

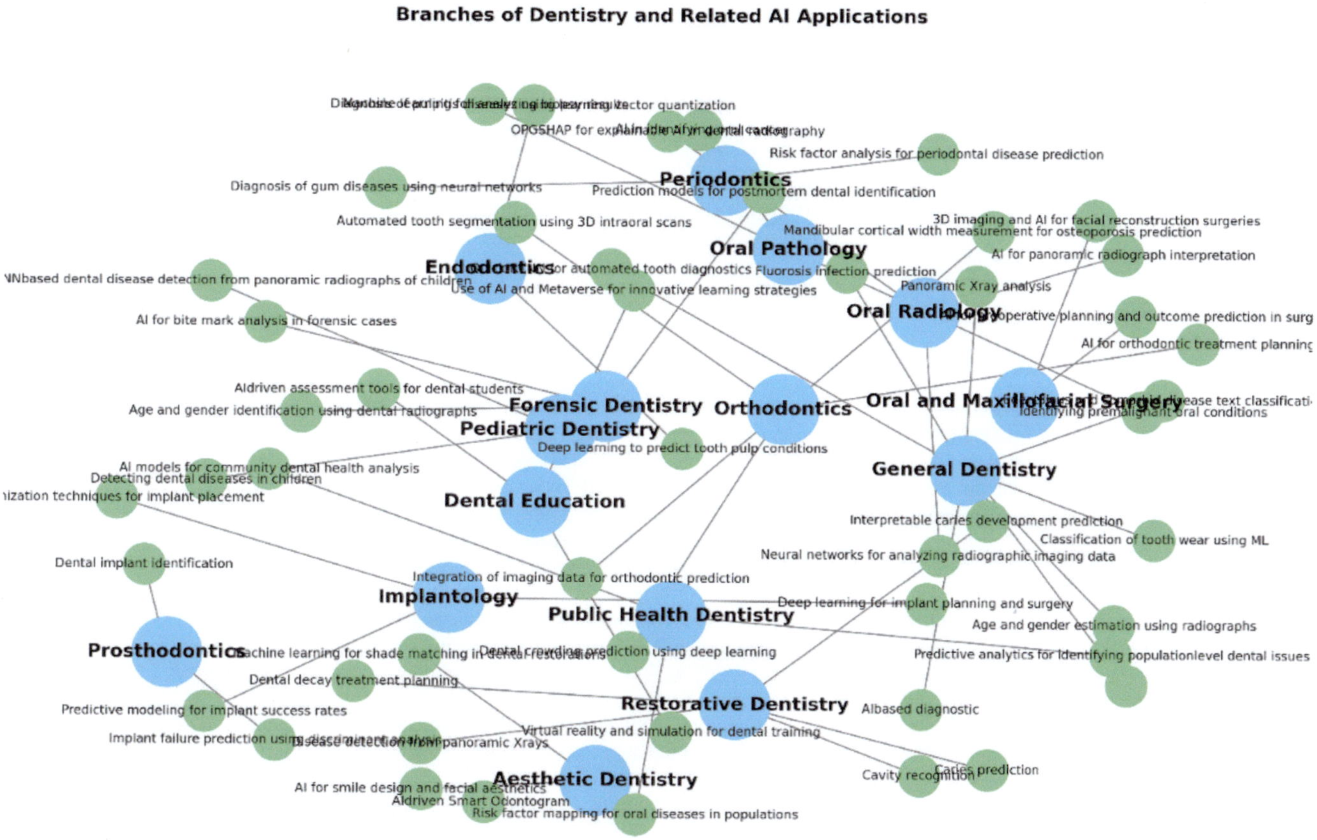


**Fig. 8.11** AI-powered operations in various branches of dentistry

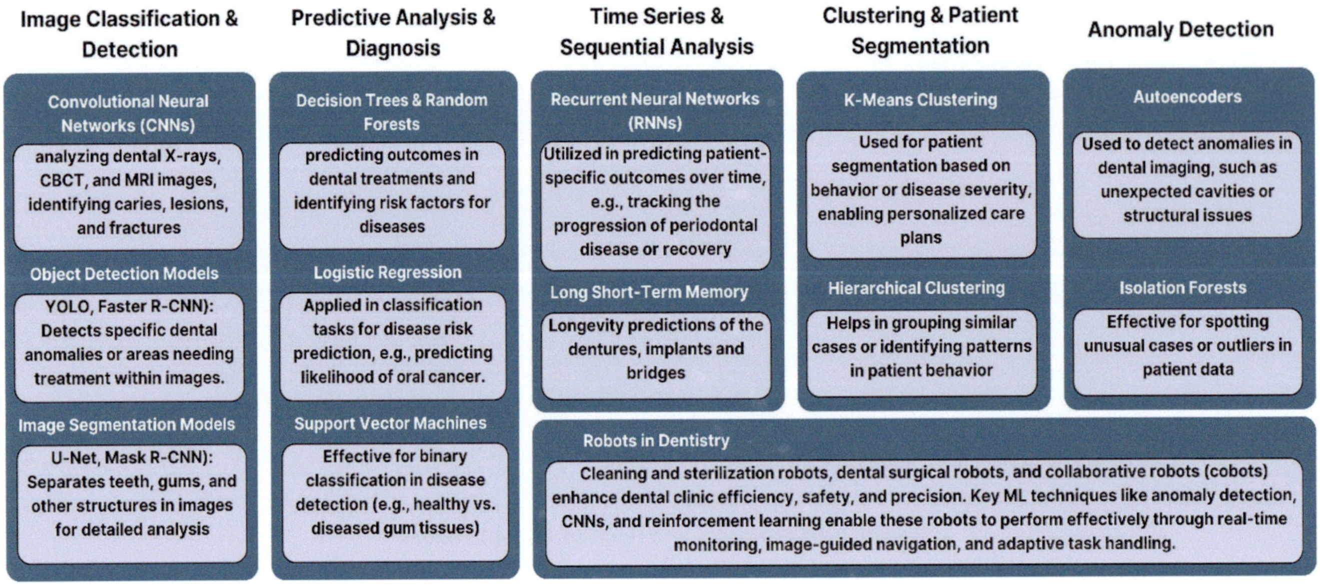


**Fig. 8.12** ML techniques used in modern dentistry

**Acknowledgements** This work was carried out in MedTech lab, IIT Kanpur which is supported by Biotechnology Industry Research Assistance Council, under National Biopharma Mission of the Department of Biotechnology, India, project number BIRAC/ME/2019246.

## References

1. Mitchell DA, Mitchell L (2014) Oxford handbook of clinical dentistry. Oxford University Press, USA
2. Proffit WR, Fields HW, Sarver DM (2007) Contemporary orthodontics 4th ed. Philadelphia: Mosby
3. Ring ME (1985) Pierre fauchard and the founding of modern dentistry. J Am Dent Assoc 110(4):561–564
4. Grand view research (2023). Dental services market size, share & trends analysis report. Retrieved from https://www.grandviewresearch.com
5. Sarantopoulos P, Chen JW (2019) Emerging dental technologies: 3D printing, robotics, and AI. Dent Today 38(11):58–64
6. Migliorati M, Signoriello A, Gherlone E (2019) The challenges of integrating AI and robotics in dental practices. J Dent Technol 27(3):45–51
7. Murphy DP, Mays KA (2021) Collaborative robotics in dentistry: emerging applications. Robot Biomimetrics 23(2):156–165
8. Krishnan A, Patel M (2022) AI and cobots: reshaping the future of dentistry. Int J Med Robot 18(4):e2389
9. Gupta S, Agarwal P (2020) The role of MedTech labs in dental advancements. J Med Devices Technol 34(7):190–205
10. Kumar V, Singh D (2022) MedTech labs and the development of collaborative robots in dentistry. Int Dent J 72(6):330–336
11. Vashisht R, Sharma A, Kiran T, Jolly SS, Brar PK, Puri JV (2024) Artificial intelligence in dentistry—A scoping review. J Oral Maxillofac Surg Med Pathol 36(4):579–592. https://doi.org/10.1016/j.ajoms.2024.04.009
12. Patil S, Nirkhi S, Kurumbanshi S, Sonawane S (2024) 1 evaluation of adaptive algorithms for recognition of cavities in dentistry. In: Machine learning methods for signal, image and speech processing, River Publishers, pp 1–22. Accessed Sept 18 2024. [Online]. Available: https://ieeexplore.ieee.org/document/9653945
13. Montenegro RD, Oliveira ALI, Cabral GG, Katz CRT, Rosenblatt A (2008) A comparative study of machine learning techniques for caries prediction. In: 2008 20th IEEE international conference on tools with artificial intelligence, Dayton, OH, USA: IEEE, pp 477–481. https://doi.org/10.1109/ICTAI.2008.138

# Cardiac Digital Twins—Computational Approaches for Personalized Arrhythmia Care

9

Ketan Rajawat

**Abstract**

Cardiac arrhythmias, including ventricular tachyarrhythmias and atrial fibrillation (AF), are major contributors to global mortality, with AF alone affecting over 45 million individuals and accounting for a significant portion of ischemic stroke cases. Current treatment approaches are limited by a lack of personalization, failing to address individual variability in arrhythmia mechanisms and risk factors. Precision cardiology seeks to overcome these limitations by tailoring therapies to each patient, made possible through advances in patient-specific data acquisition, such as genetic markers and advanced imaging. Recent innovations in digital twin technology offer promising strides toward this goal by enabling the creation of detailed, virtual heart models. These models simulate individualized cardiac function, providing a platform to predict arrhythmias more accurately and to test therapeutic interventions, such as ablation, in a simulated environment. This review explores the development and application of digital twins in cardiac electrophysiology, emphasizing their potential to enhance arrhythmia management by enabling more precise, personalized treatments. With the advancement of digital twin technologies, cardiac electrophysiology is poised for transformative progress in arrhythmia care.

**Keywords**

Computational methods · Cardiac electrophysiology · Image segmentation · Inverse problems

## 9.1 Introduction

Cardiac arrhythmias remain one of the primary contributors to global mortality and morbidity [1]. Ventricular tachyarrhythmias, for instance, are a major cause of sudden cardiac arrest (SCA), which accounts for nearly half of all cardiovascular-related deaths [2]. Similarly, atrial fibrillation (AF) impacts more than 45 million people worldwide and is a leading cause of ischemic strokes, responsible for 20–30% of cases. AF is also associated with a high rate of hospitalizations and a significantly increased risk of mortality [3]. Although advancements in diagnostic and treatment methods have been made, current strategies for managing cardiac arrhythmias often fall short of preventing these serious outcomes.

A key limitation of existing antiarrhythmic therapies is their generalized approach, which fails to consider the individual variability in risk factors and mechanisms of arrhythmia. This has spurred growing interest in the emerging field of precision cardiology, which aims to customize treatments for each patient to improve effectiveness while minimizing adverse effects. The rise of precision cardiology is made possible by advances in acquiring detailed patient-specific data, such as genetic information, biomarkers, and sophisticated imaging techniques. Yet, the challenge lies in effectively integrating this vast data into actionable clinical strategies [4].

Recent developments in digital twins have opened new possibilities for achieving the goals of precision cardiology. A digital twin is a highly detailed, individualized virtual model of a patient's heart, constructed from imaging techniques like MRI

K. Rajawat (✉)
Department of Electrical Engineering, IIT Kanpur, Kanpur, India
e-mail: ketan@iitk.ac.in



S. Verma (ed.), *Technology and Innovation in Medical Sciences*, IITK Directions 7,
https://doi.org/10.1007/978-981-96-8606-3_9

or CT. These models capture critical anatomical features, such as scar tissue that forms post-heart attack, and can simulate the heart's electrical activity, especially in areas affected by scarring. By doing so, digital twins allow for more accurate predictions of arrhythmias and offer a platform for physicians to test different treatment approaches, such as ablation, in a simulated environment before applying them to the patient in real life [5].

This review aims to provide a thorough exploration of digital twins within the realm of cardiac electrophysiology. We will provide the necessary background on cardiac electrophysiology, discuss the development of digital twins, their use in managing arrhythmia, and the challenges and opportunities they present. Through this discussion, we hope to highlight the transformative potential of digital twins in offering more individualized, precise treatments for arrhythmia, ultimately advancing the field of cardiac electrophysiology.

## 9.2 Background

The heart's ability to pump blood effectively depends on a well-timed sequence of electrical impulses that coordinate the heart muscle's contraction and relaxation. This electrical activity is essential for maintaining a regular heartbeat, allowing the heart to function as the circulatory system's pump.

### 9.2.1 Heart's Electrical System

The heart's electrical system is made up of special cells and structures that generate and send out electrical impulses. The main parts of this system are depicted in Fig. 9.1 and described here:

1. **Sinoatrial (SA) Node**: Located in the right atrium, the SA node is the heart's natural pacemaker. This node is a specialized cluster of cells that exhibits automaticity, meaning they possess the ability to depolarize at their own intrinsic rate without relying on signals from other heart cells [6]. It generates electrical impulses that start each heartbeat, producing signals 60–100 times per minute under normal conditions [7]
2. **Atrioventricular (AV) Node**: Positioned between the atria and the ventricles, the AV node acts as a relay station. It delays the electrical impulse slightly, allowing the atria to contract and push blood into the ventricles before the ventricles contract. The intrinsic rate of AV node is 40 to 60 beats per minute [8]
3. **Bundle of His**: This bundle of fibers conducts electrical impulses from the AV node down to the ventricles. It splits into the right and left bundle branches, which conduct the impulses to the respective ventricles.

**Fig. 9.1** Anatomy of the electrical system of the heart

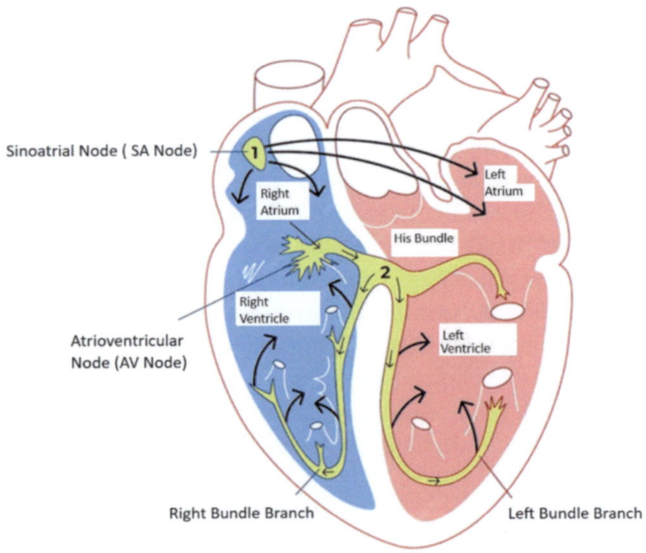

4. **Purkinje Fibers**: These specialized fibers spread throughout the ventricles, ensuring the rapid and coordinated spread of the electrical impulse, leading to efficient ventricular contraction [6]

### 9.2.2 Sequence of Electrical Activation

The sequence of electrical activation is as follows:

1. **Initiation at the SA Node**: The electrical impulse starts at the SA node, creating an action potential that spreads through the atria's walls, causing them to contract and push blood into the ventricles.
2. **Propagation to the AV Node**: The impulse travels through the atrial myocardium to the AV node. The AV node delays the impulse, allowing the ventricles time to fill with blood from the atria.
3. **Conduction through the Bundle of His and Bundle Branches**: The impulse moves quickly from the AV node to the Bundle of His and then travels down the right and left bundle branches into the ventricles.
4. **Distribution through Purkinje Fibers**: The impulse spreads through the Purkinje fibers to the ventricular myocardium, causing the ventricles to contract almost simultaneously, pumping blood out of the heart to the lungs and the rest of the body.

The precise timing of these electrical impulses ensures that the atria and ventricles contract in a coordinated manner, which is crucial for efficiently pumping blood and maintaining a regular heartbeat. The electrical impulses trigger the contraction of heart muscle cells through a process called depolarization, where the electrical charge inside the cells changes, leading to muscle contraction. After contraction, the heart muscle cells return to their resting state through repolarization, preparing them for the next impulse and contraction [9].

#### 9.2.2.1 Normal and Abnormal Heart Rhythms

In a healthy heart, the SA node sets the pace, and the electrical impulses follow the normal conduction pathway, resulting in a regular and synchronized heartbeat known as normal sinus rhythm. However, if there is a disruption in the generation or conduction of electrical impulses, arrhythmias can occur. These range from harmless conditions like premature beats to serious ones like ventricular tachycardia or fibrillation, which can be life-threatening [10].

It might be instructive to compare the electrical system of the heart with that of an electrical circuit in an engineering system. The pumping action of the heart relies on a series of precisely timed electrical impulses that ensure the heart muscles contract and relax in a coordinated sequence. The SA node acts as the primary clock generator, initiating electrical signals that trigger each heartbeat. These signals travel through a network of pathways, including the AV node, which functions like a delay circuit to ensure proper timing between the atria and ventricles. The Bundle of His and Purkinje fibers act as the conductive wires, distributing the impulses throughout the heart to ensure synchronized contractions. Just as in any electronic system, if the timing or conduction of these electrical signals is disrupted, the system (heart) can malfunction, leading to arrhythmias. Understanding the heart's electrical system in this way highlights the importance of precise timing and coordination for efficient operation.

#### 9.2.2.2 Scar Formation and Cardiac Arrhythmia

Scar tissue in the heart, known as myocardial fibrosis, can result from various conditions, with myocardial infarction (heart attack) being the primary cause [11]. During a myocardial infarction, blocked coronary arteries reduce blood flow to part of the heart muscle, causing cells to die. The body's repair process replaces these dead cells with fibrous scar tissue, which lacks the contractile properties of healthy heart muscle and can disrupt the heart's ability to pump effectively. This scarring can also interfere with the heart's electrical pathways, leading to arrhythmias such as ventricular tachycardia (VT) and ventricular fibrillation (VF). Likewise, scarring in the atria can cause atrial fibrillation (AF). Whereas the occurrence of *ventricular arrhythmia* can lead to cardiac arrest and *sudden cardiac death* [12].

##### Ventricular Tachycardia (VT)

Ventricular tachycardia (VT) is a cardiac arrhythmia where the heart's lower chambers beat rapidly, often over 100 times per minute, which can be life-threatening. The areas of slow conduction around scar tissue create conditions for electrical signals to loop back upon themselves, creating a continuous cycle of stimulation. This re-entry can occur in the ventricles, leading to the rapid and repetitive activation of the heart muscle, resulting in VT. As a result, patients often feel their heart racing or pounding in their chest. The rapid heart rate can lead to inadequate blood flow to the brain, causing dizziness or a feeling of light-headedness [7].

#### Ventricular Fibrillation (VF)

Ventricular fibrillation (VF) is one of the most severe arrhythmias linked to myocardial fibrosis, sometimes triggered by VT. In VF, the electrical activity in the ventricles becomes chaotic, causing the ventricles to quiver rather than contract in a coordinated manner. This leads to an immediate and severe decrease in the heart's ability to pump blood, resulting in a rapid loss of consciousness and, if not treated promptly, sudden cardiac death. VF is a medical emergency that requires immediate defibrillation to restore a normal heart rhythm and save the patient's life.

#### Atrial Fibrillation (AF)

Atrial fibrillation (AF), another common arrhythmia associated with myocardial fibrosis, involves erratic electrical impulses in the atria, the heart's upper chambers. These irregular impulses can cause the atria to quiver instead of contracting effectively, leading to an irregular and often rapid heartbeat. Patients with AF may experience palpitations, fatigue, shortness of breath, and an increased risk of stroke. Both VT and AF highlight the critical impact of myocardial fibrosis on the heart's electrical system and overall function [13].

VTs are a major cause of sudden cardiac arrest (SCA) and subsequent sudden cardiac death, which represents 50% of all cardiovascular deaths [2, 14]).Similarly, atrial fibrillation (AF) affects more than 45 million people worldwide and is associated with 20–30% of all ischemic strokes, a 10–40% annual hospitalization rate, and a 1.5–3.5-fold increased risk of death [3].

### 9.2.3 Treatment Options

Medications are typically the first line of treatment for arrhythmias like ventricular tachycardia (VT) and atrial fibrillation (AF), but their efficacy varies significantly among individuals. The limited efficacy of medications in the treatment of arrhythmia can be attributed to the use of a one-size-fits-most approach that ignores the diversity in arrhythmogenic risk and mechanisms [7]. For instance, antiarrhythmic drugs like beta-blockers or calcium channel blockers are prescribed broadly and provide symptomatic treatment by reducing the heart rate and blood pressure. These drugs to not address the root cause of arrhythmia and target the entire heart and cardiovascular system. The drugs are ineffective, for instance, for patients with abnormal electrical pathways due to extensive scarring.

An Implantable Cardioverter-Defibrillator (ICD) is a device implanted in the chest to monitor and correct life-threatening arrhythmias by delivering electrical shocks. The implantation procedure involves placing the device under the skin near the collarbone and threading wires through the veins into the heart. Despite their effectiveness, ICDs are not commonly used in India due to high costs, limited accessibility, and the challenge of regular follow-up care. Additionally, the current criteria for ICD implantation, particularly the left ventricular ejection fraction (LVEF) threshold of $\leq$ 40%40, may not adequately identify all patients who could benefit from the device [15].

Catheter ablation, specifically radiofrequency (RF) ablation, is a treatment for ventricular tachycardia (VT) that involves delivering energy to the heart tissue to destroy its ability to conduct abnormal electrical signals. This procedure aims to disrupt the abnormal electrical waves that sustain VT, offering the possibility of a permanent cure. However, the success rate for eliminating infarct-related VT with ablation is modest, ranging from 50 to 88% [16], while post-ablation recurrence rates remain around 25–50%.

In catheter ablation, mapping the electrical activity of the heart involves creating a detailed map of the heart's electrical signals. Coarse maps may be created using non-invasive methods like ECGs. However, higher resolution maps can only be obtained invasively via electro-anatomical mapping, which involves inserting a catheter equipped with electrodes into the heart to collect electrical data from various points [17]. Additionally, this process often involves limited spatial sampling, which means that only specific, and sometimes sparse, areas of the heart are analyzed. Limited spatial sampling can result in incomplete or imprecise maps, making it difficult to identify the critical pathways that are responsible for propagating VT [18].

During the ablation procedure, patients may experience hemodynamic stress, which strains the heart and circulatory system, affecting stability and heart performance, and complicating the identification of abnormal electrical pathways. Correlating electrical maps with the heart's complex three-dimensional anatomy can be challenging, as these maps are two-dimensional representations, potentially leading to errors in targeting areas for ablation. The intricate three-dimensional pathways of

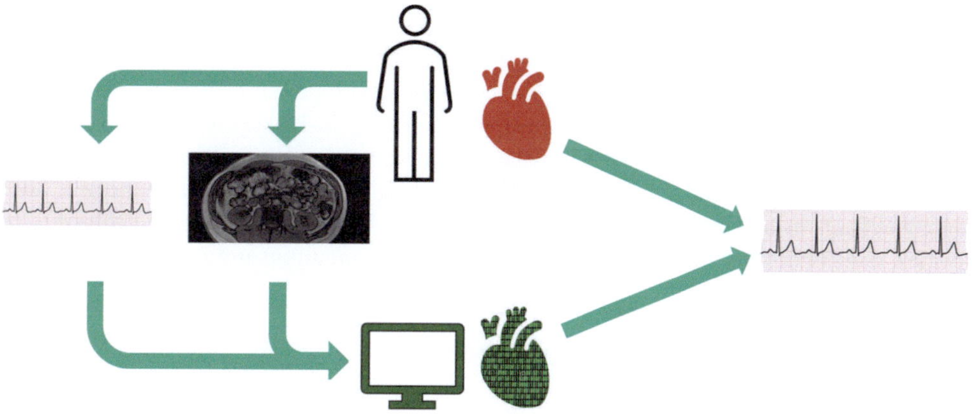

**Fig. 9.2** Cardiac digital twin to enable personalized in-silico cardiology

electrical impulses around the infarct zone are difficult to reconstruct accurately, often resulting in imprecise ablation targets and unnecessarily large lesions. This can extend the procedure duration to 4–12 h, increasing the risk of complications, radiation exposure, and damage to healthy heart tissue, which can negatively impact heart function.

## 9.3 Digital Twins for Treating Arrhythmia

**Precision cardiology** is an innovative approach to cardiovascular care that tailors diagnosis, treatment, and prevention strategies to the individual characteristics of each patient. This field leverages advanced technologies and methodologies, such as genetic testing, 'omics' (including genomics, proteomics, and metabolomics), biomarkers, and detailed imaging techniques, to gather comprehensive patient-specific information. By integrating these diverse data sources, precision cardiology aims to understand the unique factors contributing to a patient's cardiovascular condition.

Unlike traditional cardiology, which often employs generalized treatments based on broad population averages, precision cardiology focuses on the unique genetic, molecular, and environmental factors influencing each patient's health. This personalized approach enhances the accuracy of diagnoses, optimizes treatment efficacy, and reduces the risk of adverse effects.

**Digital twins**, which are virtual models of a patient's heart created using specific genetic, biological, and physiological data, represent a highly personalized approach to treating arrhythmias as depicted in Fig. 9.2. These digital replicas simulate the cardiac electrophysiology of an individual's heart, allowing clinicians to predict how the heart will respond to various treatments. In the modern electrophysiology (EP) workplace, digital twins fit seamlessly by providing detailed simulations that guide precise interventions, such as catheter ablation, without subjecting patients to unnecessary risk. Digital twins are revolutionary in their ability to integrate vast amounts of patient-specific data, producing highly accurate and individualized treatment plans that enhance outcomes and minimize adverse effects, marking a significant advancement over traditional one-size-fits-all approaches. For example, a digital twin can help determine the most effective antiarrhythmic drug for a particular patient or guide the precise targeting of ablation therapy for those with complex arrhythmias. By using digital twins, doctors can personalize treatments to each patient's unique needs, improving outcomes and reducing the likelihood of adverse effects [19].

## 9.4 Computational Electrophysiology

Computational electrophysiology involves the use of mathematical models and computer simulations to understand and predict the electrical behavior of biological cells, particularly in the context of cardiac functions. By creating virtual representations of cellular activities, researchers can study complex phenomena such as action potentials, ion channel dynamics, and arrhythmias in a controlled, repeatable environment. This interdisciplinary field bridges biology, mathematics, and computer science, providing critical insights that can drive advancements in medical treatments, drug development, and our fundamental understanding of physiological processes.

The field of computational electrophysiology was sparked by Hodgkin and Huxley's groundbreaking work in 1952 on the squid giant axon, which demonstrated that the experimentally observed action potential could be quantitatively reproduced using an electrical circuit model [20]. This led to the development of various mathematical models for neural and cardiac electrophysiology. In 1962, Denis Noble adapted the Hodgkin-Huxley equations to study the cardiac action potential, paving the way for more specialized models like the Beeler-Reuter model in 1977 [21]. Advances in experimental techniques, such as the patch-clamp method and molecular biology tools, further refined these models, allowing for the inclusion of detailed ionic mechanisms and intracellular processes. Over the decades, models have evolved to represent different cardiac regions, species, and conditions, culminating in patient-specific simulations used in clinical settings.

### 9.4.1 Example Box: Courtemanche Model

The Courtemanche model is a mathematical representation used to describe the electrical activity of cardiac cells, particularly the atrial myocytes. It uses differential equations to model the ionic currents and how they contribute to the action potential (AP) of the cell.

In this context, the **Membrane potential** $V_m$ describes the voltage difference across a cell's membrane. For this purpose, one may imagine the cell membrane as an insulating layer, similar to the plastic coating around a wire. It separates the inside of the cell (cytoplasm) from the outside environment (extracellular fluid).

While in electronics, we consider electrons as charge carriers, in biological systems, the charge is carried by ions such as sodium $\mathrm{Na}^+$, calcium $\mathrm{Ca}^+$, potassium $\mathrm{K}^+$ and Chloride $\mathrm{Cl}^-$. The ion channels in the membranes act like resistors or switches in a circuit, controlling the flow of ions in and out of the cell. In cardiac cells, the resting membrane potential is typically around -85mV due to difference in the abundance of positive and negative ions inside and outside the cell. As ions flow through various switches, the change in the membrane potential $\frac{\mathrm{d}V_m}{\mathrm{dt}}$ is governed by these ionic currents and the capacitance of the membrane ($C_m$):

$$C_m \frac{\mathrm{d}V_m}{\mathrm{dt}} = -(I_{\mathrm{Na}} + I_K + I_{\mathrm{Ca}} + I_{\mathrm{other}} + I_{\mathrm{stim}})$$

where $I_{\mathrm{Na}}$, $I_K$, $I_{\mathrm{Ca}}$, and $I_{\mathrm{other}}$ represent the various ionic currents while $I_{\mathrm{stim}}$ represents the stimulus current. These current values are again functions of $V_m$ and may be described by differential equations of their own. As an example, we have that $I_{\mathrm{Na}} = g_{\mathrm{Na}} m^3 h (V_m - E_{\mathrm{Na}})$ where

- $g_{\mathrm{Na}}$ is the maximum conductance and $E_{\mathrm{Na}}$ is the reversal potential, both of which are known constants
- The gating variables are defined as sigmoidal functions that either close to 0 or close to 1, depending on $V_m$:

$$m = \frac{1}{1 + \exp\left(-\frac{(V_m + 40\,mV)}{10}\right)} \text{ and } h = \frac{1}{1 + \exp\left(\frac{(V_m + 60\,mV)}{10}\right)}$$

where $V_m$ is expressed in mV. We see that the activation gate $m$ is negligible in the resting state (when $V_m \approx -80\,\mathrm{mV}$) but becomes significant upon depolarization, i.e., when $V_m$ increases much beyond $-40$ mV. On the other hand, the inactivation gate $h$ is close to 1 in the resting state but decreases to 0 when $V_m$ is much beyond $-20$ mV.

Given these equations, let us try to understand the evolution of $V_m$ intuitively. At the resting state, $m \approx 0$ and $h \approx 1$. When stimulus is applied, $V_m$ increases slightly, causing $m$ to increase and thus making $I_{\mathrm{Na}}$ positive. In the ODE, the value of $E_{\mathrm{Na}}$ is around 50 mV, and since $V - E_{\mathrm{Na}}$ is always negative, it is evident that a positive $I_{\mathrm{Na}}$ leads to further increase in $V_m$. This creates a positive feedback loop, where the rising $V_m$ causes more sodium channels to open, further increasing $I_{\mathrm{Na}}$ and continuing the cycle of $V_m$ rising.

However, the positive feedback loop however cannot continue indefinitely and once $V_m$ goes beyond $-20$ mV, the inactivation gate $h$ starts to decrease, decreasing $I_{\mathrm{Na}}$ even when $m \approx 1$. Rising $V_m$ also increases potassium ion current $I_K$ in the opposite direction. Therefore, the membrane potential reaches a peak when the inactivation of sodium channels and the activation of potassium channels balance the depolarizing sodium current. Following this peak, the increase in $I_K$ and the inactivation of $I_{\mathrm{Na}}$ causes $V_m$ to repolarize and return toward the resting potential. The overall cycle, depicted in Fig. 9.3, lasts from 200 to 400 ms and is essential for generating the action potential that drives each heartbeat [22].

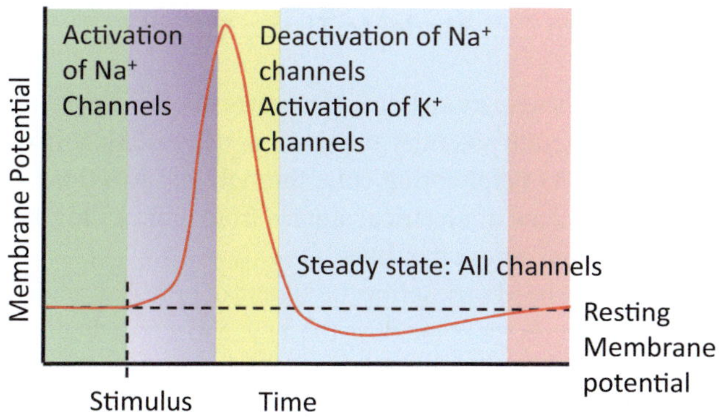


**Fig. 9.3** Adapted from Verma, Parul and Kienle, Achim and Flockerzi, Dietrich and Ramkrishna, Doraiswami. (2019). Using Bifurcation Theory for Exploring Pain. https://doi.org/10.1021/acs.iecr.9b04495

### 9.4.2 Simulating Single Cell Dynamics

The Courtemanche model is an ordinary differential equation (ODE) that describes how the membrane potential and ionic currents evolve over time within a single cell. While some ODEs can be solved analytically, the complexity of the Courtemanche model usually requires numerical methods for solutions. To this end, we may use one of the many existing algorithms, such as the Euler method, Runge–Kutta method, and the backward differentiation formula (BDF), each with its advantages and disadvantages. For instance, the Euler method is fast and requires few computations but can be inaccurate or unstable for some ODEs [23]. On the other hand, BDF is more computationally intensive but yields accurate and stable solutions. Fortunately, these algorithms have been well-studied over the past several decades and their efficient implementations are available in most commercial and open-source software packages.

### 9.4.3 Walkthrough of a Heartbeat

In the Courtemanche model of cardiac electrophysiology, the application of a stimulus by the sinoatrial (SA) node initiates a sequence of events that leads to the coordinated contraction of the heart. Here's a detailed description of what happens when the stimulus is applied by the SA node and the subsequent steps in the heart:

1. The SA node, located in the right atrium, acts as a natural pacemaker of the heart and generates an action potential spontaneously due to its automaticity. The stimulus current, modeled as a brief pulse of around 1 ms duration, causes an almost instantaneous depolarization (increase) of the membrane potential and opens the voltage-gated sodium channels, leading to an influx of $Na^+$ ions. This sets off the electrical activity and causes further increase in the membrane potential that propagates along the cardiac tissue.
2. The action potential first spreads through the atrial muscle fibers, causing the atria to contract and pushing the blood into the ventricles.
3. Simultaneously, the action potential also travels to the AV node, located at the junction of the atria and ventricles. The AV node functions as a gatekeeper, delaying the signal by approximately 0.1 s. This delay ensures the atria have sufficient time to contract fully and pump blood into the ventricles before ventricular contraction begins.
4. From the AV node, the action potential travels down the Bundle of His, which splits into the left and right bundle branches, further branching into the Purkinje fibers that spread throughout the ventricles. This system resembles a wiring network: the Bundle of His is the main transmission line, the left and right bundle branches are primary distribution wires, and the Purkinje fibers are local distribution wires, ensuring the signal is uniformly spread for synchronized contraction.
5. The action potential rapidly spreads through the Purkinje fibers, causing the ventricular muscle cells to depolarize almost simultaneously. This rapid and coordinated depolarization triggers the contraction of the ventricles, pumping blood out of the heart to the lungs (right ventricle) and the rest of the body (left ventricle) [9].

### 9.4.4 From Cell-Model to Tissue Model

The Courtemanche model only describes the ionic currents and dynamics of individual cells. Hence, it can only be used to simulate the action potential of a single cell in isolation. In cardiac tissue, when a cell becomes electrically active (depolarized), it influences its neighboring cells through gap junctions. This can be mathematically modeled using a diffusion term that describes the flow of electrical signals from areas of higher potential to areas of lower potential, facilitating the spread of the action potential across the tissue.

As we now need to describe the spread of potential across a 3D region (the cardiac tissue) and over time so we write $V_m(\mathbf{x}, t)$ where $\mathbf{x}$ is the vector containing the $x$, $y$, and $z$ coordinates for each point within the heart. We also need a conductivity tensor $\boldsymbol{\sigma}$ (which is a $3 \times 3$ matrix) that models the directional properties of the tissue, allowing for non-uniform (anisotropic) propagation of electric current along different axes. The resulting Reaction–Diffusion (RD) equation is a partial differential equation (PDE) given by

$$C_m \frac{\mathrm{d}V_m}{\mathrm{d}t} = \beta^{-1} \nabla \cdot (\boldsymbol{\sigma} \nabla V_m) - (I_{\mathrm{Na}} + I_K + I_{\mathrm{Ca}} + I_{\mathrm{other}} + I_{\mathrm{stim}})$$

where $C_m$ is the capacitance per unit area of the membrane and $\beta$ is the area of the membrane per unit volume. In this equation, the Nabla operator ($\nabla$) calculates the gradient in $x$, $y$, and $z$ directions, so that the spatial rate of change of the potential $\nabla V_m$ is a $3 \times 1$ vector with components $\frac{\mathrm{d}V_m}{\mathrm{d}x}$, $\frac{\mathrm{d}V_m}{\mathrm{d}y}$, and $\frac{\mathrm{d}V_m}{\mathrm{d}z}$. The product $\boldsymbol{\sigma} \nabla V_m$ is also a $3 \times 1$ vector but adjusts the rate of the spread according to the tissue conductivities. Finally, the divergence of this quantity, $\nabla \cdot (\boldsymbol{\sigma} \nabla V_m)$ is a scalar that measures how this adjusted rate of change is spreading out in space.

The RD model, also referred to as the monodomain model, is one of the simplest models that is reasonably accurate. More detailed and accurate models, such as the bidomain and the Reaction-Eikonal (RE) models have since been developed and widely adopted. These models are also expressed as a system of PDEs and must be solved using a numerical method, possibly using standard methods implemented in commercial software [24].

The **Finite Element Method (FEM)** begins by discretizing the spatial domain into a mesh composed of smaller, simple elements (e.g., tetrahedra). Within each element, the solution $V_m$ is approximated using basis functions, which are typically polynomials that are 1 at their corresponding node and 0 at others. This local approximation is pieced together to form the global solution. The PDE is then reformulated in a weak form by multiplying it by a test function and integrating over each element, ensuring that the residuals are minimized.

Next, the FEM involves integrating the weak form over each element to obtain local systems of linear equations. These local contributions are assembled into a global system of linear equations, with a large but sparse matrix. Boundary conditions are applied, and the system is solved using linear algebra techniques such as Gaussian elimination, LU decomposition, or iterative methods like the Conjugate Gradient. FEM effectively transforms a complex PDE into a manageable linear system, allowing for approximate solutions over complex geometries [25, 26].

### 9.4.5 Mechanistic Versus Data-Driven Models

So far, we have described the mechanistic models that simulate the electrical activity of cardiac cells and tissues based on fundamental principles of physics and biology. These models integrate experimental data with biophysical principles to enable dynamic simulations of cardiac electrophysiology at various scales, from the opening and closing of individual ion channels to the complex patterns of electrical excitation and re-excitation at the organ level. These detailed representations of ion channels, membrane potentials, and cellular interactions often use systems of differential equations derived from empirical data and theoretical considerations. For instance, similar mechanistic models have been developed to represent specific pathologies such as hypertrophic cardiomyopathy, heart failure, and atrial fibrillation, enabling multi-scale organ-level simulations to study the determinants of arrhythmia initiation and stability [27, 28]. Since the early 2000s, organ-level models based on patient-specific anatomies have been further personalized with structural remodeling derived from non-invasive imaging data, making significant real-world impacts.

The widespread availability of computational resources and the abundance of large datasets have also facilitated the development of data-driven models. In contrast to mechanistic models, data-driven models leverage large datasets and machine learning techniques to identify patterns and make predictions without necessarily understanding the underlying biological mechanisms. For example, in cardiac electrophysiology, machine learning algorithms can be trained on extensive datasets of electrocardiogram (ECG) recordings to detect and predict cardiac arrhythmias with high precision. These models can quickly process vast amounts of ECG data, identifying subtle changes indicative of potential issues such as atrial fibrillation or ventricular tachycardia. Similarly, data-driven approaches can be employed to classify different types of heartbeats or to predict the outcomes of cardiac procedures based on historical patient data [29].

However, the performance of data-driven models is heavily dependent on the quality and comprehensiveness of the training data. They often struggle to generalize beyond the specific conditions and scenarios represented in their training datasets. A model trained predominantly on data with certain types of cardiac pathologies may not perform as well when validated on data containing other conditions. This limitation means that while data-driven models can be highly effective within their training space, their predictive power diminishes when confronted with novel or less frequent cases.

In contrast, since the mechanistic models are grounded in the underlying biology and physics, they are better equipped to generalize across various scenarios, including those not explicitly represented in their initial parameter sets. For example, mechanistic models can be adapted to simulate the effects of new pharmacological agents on cardiac electrophysiology, predict the impact of genetic mutations on ion channel function, or explore the mechanisms underlying complex arrhythmias. Indeed, the generalization capabilities of mechanistic models make them valuable tools for hypothesis testing, guiding experimental design, and developing new therapeutic strategies.

## 9.5 Personalized Care via Digital Twins

A remarkable feature of mechanistic models, such as the monodomain and bidomain models is that they can be personalized with patient-specific data, such as anatomical and structural information from non-invasive imaging, to create tailored simulations that support precision medicine initiatives. This personalization paves the way for the development of "digital twins" in cardiac electrophysiology—virtual replicas of individual patients' hearts. Digital twins integrate detailed anatomical data from imaging modalities like MRI or CT scans with functional data from ECGs and other diagnostic tools, creating a comprehensive, patient-specific model that can simulate the heart's electrical activity and predict its response to various interventions.

Digital twins offer a transformative approach to cardiac care by enabling clinicians to test different treatment strategies in a virtual environment before applying them to the patient. For example, they can simulate the effects of different anti-arrhythmic drugs, ablation procedures, or implantable devices like pacemakers and defibrillators. This allows for the optimization of treatment plans, reducing the risk of adverse effects and improving patient outcomes. Recent applications of CDTs have demonstrated success in predicting the risk of sudden cardiac death in myocardial infarction patients [30], identifying ablation targets for VT [31] and AF [32], and selecting pacing sites for cardiac resynchronization therapy [33].

In clinical research, digital twins can be used to study the progression of cardiac diseases and the impact of potential new therapies. By simulating various scenarios and interventions on a digital twin, researchers can gain insights into disease mechanisms and identify promising treatment pathways more efficiently than traditional trial-and-error methods [34].

Furthermore, digital twins can facilitate personalized risk assessments [30] and preventive care. For instance, they can help identify patients at high risk of developing specific arrhythmias or other cardiac conditions based on their unique anatomical and physiological characteristics. This proactive approach enables early intervention and more targeted monitoring, potentially preventing serious cardiac events before they occur.

## 9.6 A Digital Twin for Cardiac Electrophysiology

In this section, we describe the process of building a cardiac electrophysiology digital twin as represented in Fig. 9.4. The creation of such a digital twin begins with acquiring high-resolution MRI scans, which provide detailed anatomical and structural information about the heart and surrounding tissues. These images are used to construct a three-dimensional model of the patient's heart, capturing its unique geometry and any structural abnormalities. Simultaneously, a 12-lead ECG is recorded to capture the electrical activity of the heart at that moment. This ECG data is crucial for calibrating the digital twin, ensuring that the simulated electrical activity aligns with the patient's actual cardiac function. The ECG provides information about the timing and propagation of electrical impulses across different regions of the heart, which can be used to fine-tune the model parameters.

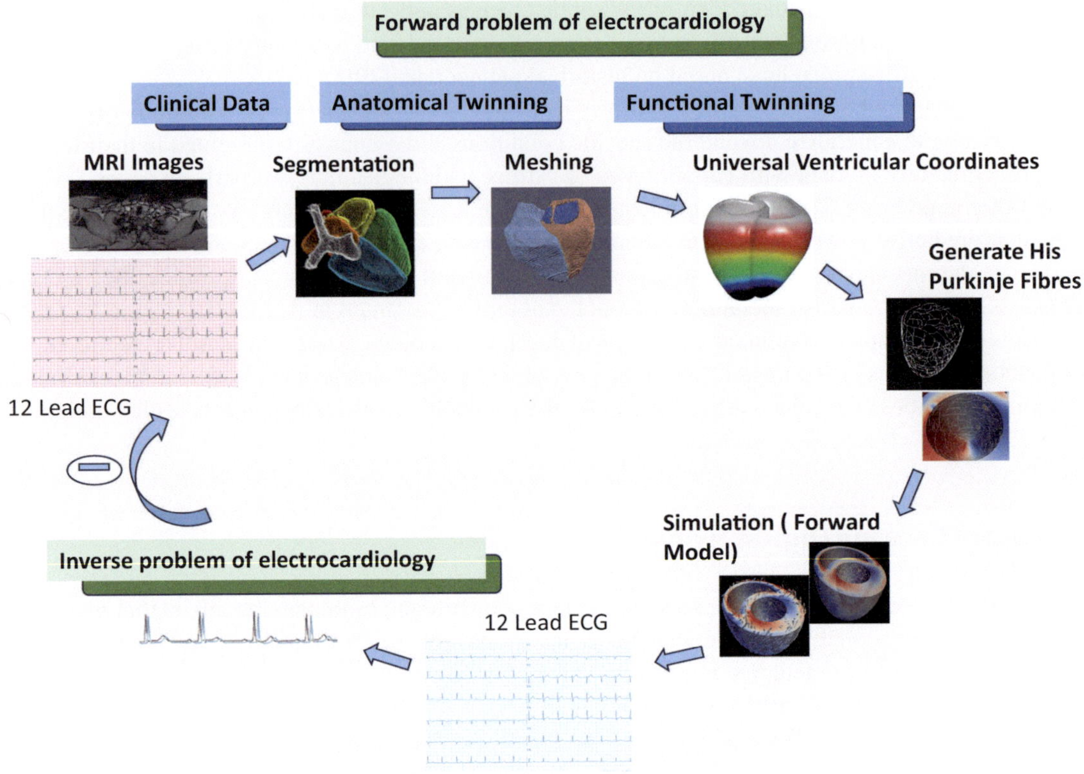


**Fig. 9.4** Overview of steps in cardiac electrophysiology simulation study

### 9.6.1 Anatomical Model

To create the anatomical model, we make use of MRI scans of the heart as well as the full torso.

1. **Segmentation:** The process begins with segmenting the heart and torso from MRI images. This involves identifying and separating different parts of the heart (the four chambers, the outer and inner walls) and surrounding structures (like aorta, lungs, and general torso tissue) from the images. Segmentation is typically performed semi-automatically using commercial software such as Seg3D, which utilizes pre-trained convolutional neural networks for this task. Any errors in the segmentation process are then manually corrected (by a trained radiologist) to ensure accuracy. Figure 9.3 shows an example of a segmented 3D image of a heart, where each segment is shown in a different color for visualization [35–37].
2. **Alignment:** Next, the segmented heart and torso images are aligned using an algorithm known as point set registration or scan matching, commonly used in autonomous robotics and self-driving cars. In the context of creating a digital twin, point set registration involves taking the segmented images of the heart and torso and precisely aligning them to ensure they are correctly positioned relative to each other [38].
3. **3D Mesh Generation:** Once the heart and torso are properly aligned, another software, such as CARPentry [39], is used to generate detailed 3D meshes of the heart and surrounding structures. It is remarked that 3D meshes are geometric representations created from segmented images, consisting of interconnected points that define the surfaces of the heart and torso structures. Unlike images that capture visual details, meshes provide precise geometric models essential for computational simulations and detailed analyses [24, 40, 41].

### 9.6.2 Universal Coordinate Systems

Human hearts are not only complex in shape but also exhibit significant variability between individuals. The relative positions of various anatomical features can differ greatly from person to person, making classical *x*-*y*-*z* coordinates insufficient for consistently and intuitively describing the heart's properties. Just as the Earth's geography requires the use of latitude, longitude, and altitude; to conveniently specify points regardless of the terrain, we need a universal coordinate system for the heart. Such a coordinate system considers the heart's natural geometry and specific anatomical landmarks, allowing for smoother and more accurate representation of data. It also facilitates the comparison of data across different heart models by ensuring consistent positional references, regardless of individual variations in heart shape and size.

Several universal coordinate systems have been proposed in the literature. Universal Ventricular Coordinates (UVC) provide a systematic way to describe the position within the ventricles of the heart using four parameters: $\lambda$ (lambda), $\rho$ (rho), $\phi$ (phi), and $\nu$ (nu). To compute these coordinates, the user needs to input specific points on the heart: an epicardial apex point, an LV endocardial point, an RV septal point, and points at the ventricular base. The process involves separating the ventricles and solving Laplace's equation under specific boundary conditions. The $\lambda$ coordinate represents the distance from the apex to the base, $\rho$ represents the transmural distance from the endocardium to the epicardium, $\phi$ represents the circumferential rotation around the long axes of the ventricles, and $\nu$ distinguishes between the left and right ventricles. By defining these coordinates, the UVC system enables consistent and accurate mapping and transfer of data between different heart models, facilitating more precise and reliable electrophysiology simulations [42, 43].

### 9.6.3 His-Purkinje System

Recall that the His-Purkinje fibers are specialized conducting fibers in the heart responsible for distributing electrical signals throughout the myocardium. These fibers are assigned a significantly higher conduction velocity than the surrounding tissue to simulate their effects on electrical signaling. Unfortunately, the His-Purkinje system is usually not visible on standard-resolution MRI or CT scans because its fibers are very small and lack enough contrast from the surrounding heart muscle. Additionally, there is limited knowledge about its precise structure and variations within the human population. In recent years, researchers have utilized procedural network generation algorithms, such as fractal trees, to create models of the HPS. Remarkably, although these generated fiber meshes are randomized and not anatomically accurate, they are sufficient for electrophysiological simulations. HPS generation algorithms have been validated in clinical settings in [44]. By comparing simulated and measured electro-anatomical maps of local activation times, with most errors under 10 ms, demonstrating high accuracy.

Additionally, the computational models also allow for automated personalization, where the algorithm parameters can be tuned to minimize the discrepancies between the simulated and measured ECGs, further enhancing precision [45].

### 9.6.4 Forward Electrophysiological Modeling

Before carrying out the simulations, each node within the mesh must be assigned certain tissue-specific properties, such as conduction velocities and conductivities that will subsequently be used by the forward model to propagate the electrical signals at the SA node. However, most of these parameters are unknown and cannot be measured non-invasively. There are two main approaches to address this challenge (a) using typical values that still yield reasonably accurate ECGs or (b) personalizing the values by tuning them to better match the ECGs. For simplicity, let us consider the first case, where typical parameter values are used. We will revisit the process of personalization in the next section.

Having set the parameter values and selected the appropriate forward modeling paradigm, i.e., one of RD Monodomain [46]., RD Bidomain [24], RE Lead Field [45], etc., it remains to solve the constituent PDEs in an appropriate software. While a large number of solvers support solving these PDEs, some of the popular ones that are currently in use include OpenCARP [47] and Ansys [48]. Of these, OpenCARP is an open-source cardiac electrophysiology simulator which has its roots in the Cardiac Arrhythmia Research Package (CARP) platform developed in early 2000s (Fig. 9.5).

On the other hand, Ansys is a general-purpose engineering simulation software and features add-ons that can be used for cardiac electrophysiology simulations. The output of such a simulation is a waveform representing the electrical signal, at each point on the heart and torso. The output can be used to visualize the propagation of the electrical signals in three dimensions, as depicted in Fig. 9.5 Here, each sub figure shows the snapshot of electrical activity at different instants of time, while the color encodes the voltage level. Alternatively, one can extract the electrical waveforms at different points on the torso, resulting in the simulated ECGs [45].

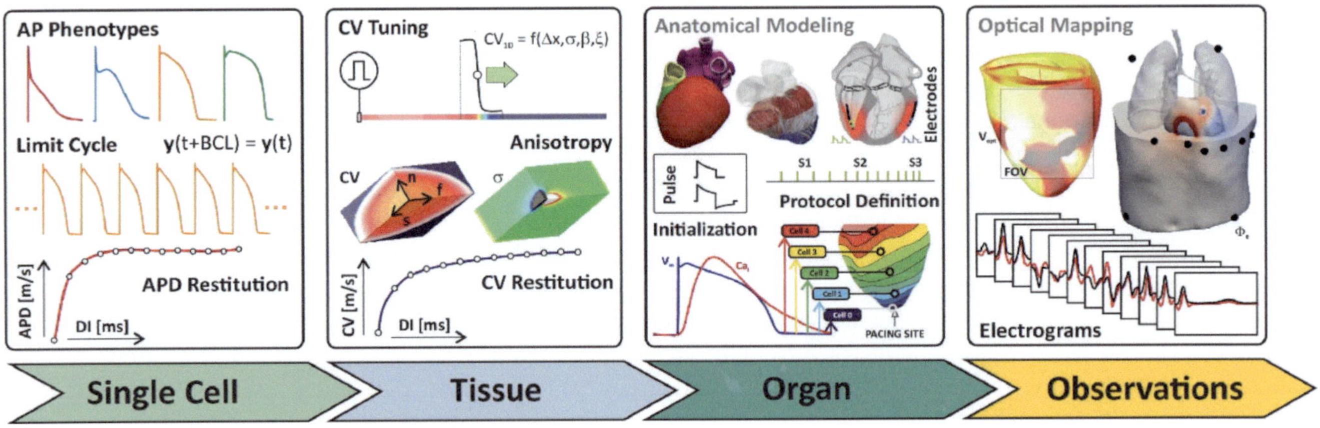


**Fig. 9.5** Steps used in OpenCARP see: https://opencarp.org/

### 9.6.5 Inverse Electrophysiological Modeling

Inverse modeling, or personalization, aims to improve the accuracy of electrophysiological predictions by adjusting key model parameters to reflect the unique characteristics of each individual. Personalization is well-motivated for model parameters that are either unknown (e.g., conductivities and conduction velocities) or artificial (e.g., parameters associated with the procedurally generated HPS). The process of personalization involves solving an optimization problem and is captured by the following pseudo-code:

Set all parameters to their typical values.

**Repeat**:

1. Run the forward model to generate simulated ECGs
2. Compare the simulated ECGs with the measured ECGs
3. Select a new set of parameters that are likely to reduce the error between the measured and simulated ECGs.

A key aspect of this process is that the forward modeling must be repeated for many different sets of potential parameters. The selection of parameters likely to reduce error in subsequent iterations is typically handled by an optimization algorithm [45].

Various optimization algorithms can be used for this purpose and here we discuss a few.

**Bayesian Optimization** is a black-box optimization method that builds a probabilistic model of the objective function and uses it to explore parameter space efficiently. Bayesian optimization has been widely used in similar settings and can be tuned to achieve the correct trade-off between the number of iterations and minimum error it achieves [49]. There also exist other deterministic black-box methods, such as **Nelder-Mead**, that can systematically explore the parameter space based on the error performance of previous parameter sets [50].

Alternatively, one can also use the classical **gradient descent** or its variants, especially if the error varies smoothly with the variation in the parameters. For this class of algorithms however, the gradients must be calculated numerically or by modifying the simulation framework itself using techniques such as the complex step method [51].

Each of these algorithms have their advantages and disadvantages, and it is best to try multiple approaches on a large number of different problems before selecting the algorithm of choice.

## 9.7 State-Of-The-Art in Cardiac Digital Twins

Digital twins, though promising for use in cardiac electrophysiology and arrhythmia management, have yet to become common in clinical practice.

One of the seminal works to utilize digital twins for predicting the risk of SCA was [30]. The work considered a cohort of 41 patients suffering from a heart condition called ischemic cardiomyopathy, where the blood flow to the heart is reduced. The work showed that digital twins constructed using MRI scans were better at predicting SCA risk than the traditional approach that only targets patients with reduced left-ventricular ejection fraction.

Arevalo's work was one of the first to utilize cardiac electrophysiology simulations for risk stratification. It also demonstrated that since simulations are accurate enough to predict arrhythmias, they can also be used to test how different treatment approaches might work before actually performing them on a patient. It sparked a number of retrospective studies, where the simulations were tested on data from patients who had already undergone treatment in order to compare the efficacy of the simulation-based approaches with the state-of-the-art approaches used by doctors. The studies considered cases of VT [16, 52]), AF [53], as well as inherited arrhythmia conditions [54]. These studies showed potential for guiding treatments like catheter ablation, where doctors burn small areas of heart tissue to prevent arrhythmias. There have also been small prospective studies where digital twins were used to guide the personalized ablation in VT [31] and AF [32].

One of the first larger-scale studies tested digital twin-guided ablation in 108 patients with AF [55]. The patients were divided into two groups: one got routine treatment, and the other received treatment guided by simulations based on their heart's 3D model. Although the study showed it was possible to use these models to plan ablation, there was no significant improvement in outcomes compared to standard treatment, even though the simulation-guided group had more extensive procedures.

However, a more recent, larger study with 170 patients showed that using these digital models to guide treatment did improve outcomes for people with persistent AF [56]. Another ongoing study is comparing routine ablation with simulation-guided ablation, using MRI scans to create patient-specific heart models [32].

## 9.8 Challenges and Opportunities

Despite the advances and studies mentioned earlier, no clinical trials have yet been registered for using digital twins in managing ventricular arrhythmias or for preventing sudden cardiac death. While technology shows promise, but it is still early in its development, and more research is needed before it becomes a routine part of arrhythmia management in hospitals. Below we list a few challenges.

**Reproducibility and model sharing**: Many different research groups create digital twin frameworks using custom, often poorly documented code. This lack of standardized sharing hinders reproducibility and validation across the field, even though some platforms like Myokit [57] and OpenCARP [47] have improved model sharing.

**Limitations of Imaging for Personalization**: Current non-invasive imaging methods like CT and CMR, while useful, have limitations such as poor resolution and overestimation of scar tissue (fibrosis). These issues make it difficult to accurately map all details of a patient's heart, impacting the precision of digital twins [58].

**Incomplete Personalization of Electrical Properties**: While imaging helps map heart structure, the personalization of electrical properties (e.g., by tuning the unknown parameters such as conductivity) is less advanced. Standard ECGs provide limited spatial data, and while non-invasive mapping (ECGI) can help, it lacks full accuracy and detail [45].

**Dynamic Data and Time-Varying Risks**: Most digital twins use static data captured at one moment in time, but the heart's electrical system and arrhythmia risks change dynamically. Methods for integrating time-varying data from wearables or ongoing tests are still in development [59].

**Complexity of Large-Scale Clinical Trials**: High-quality clinical trials (RCTs) are necessary to prove that digital twins improve treatment outcomes. These trials are complex, expensive, and take time to organize, requiring collaboration between clinicians and researchers [60].

**Implementation Challenges in Clinical Practice**: Even if clinical trials are successful, significant efforts are needed to standardize workflows, automate processes, and ensure that digital twins can be integrated into everyday clinical practice without causing disruptions.

**Cost-effectiveness and Feasibility**: Digital twins must not only show clinical benefits but also prove to be cost-effective and feasible for treating large numbers of patients in real-world healthcare settings to gain widespread adoption.

**Acknowledgements** We extend our gratitude to our collaborators A. Kulkarni, B. Kuiri, R. Dash, N. Sawant, and K. Rajpurohit for their dedicated contributions to the technical aspects of the Cardiac Digital Twin project. We also thank Profs. K. Muralidhar, T. Sandhan, P. Bagade, and B. V.

Rathish Kumar for their invaluable guidance and several insightful suggestions throughout the project. Special thanks to Dr. A. Singh for their assistance in editing, figure preparation, and reference management for this manuscript. Additionally, we thank IIT Kanpur for funding the project.

## References

1. Timmis A, Vardas P, Townsend N et al (2022) European society of cardiology: cardiovascular disease statistics 2021. Eur Heart J J43:716–799
2. Zeppenfeld K, Tfelt-Hansen J, De Riva M, Winkel BG, Behr ER, Blom NA, Volterrani M (2022) ESC guidelines for the management of patients with ventricular arrhythmias and the prevention of sudden cardiac death: Developed by the task force for the management of patients with ventricular arrhythmias and the prevention of sudden cardiac death of the European Society of Cardiology (ESC) Endorsed by the Association for European Paediatric and Congenital Cardiology (AEPC). Eur Heart J 43(40):3997–4126
3. Hindricks G, Potpara T, Dagres N, Arbelo E, Bax JJ, Blomström-Lundqvist C, Watkins CL (2021) 2020 ESC Guidelines for the diagnosis and management of atrial fibrillation developed in collaboration with the European Association for Cardio-Thoracic Surgery (EACTS) The task force for the diagnosis and management of atrial fibrillation of the European Society of Cardiology (ESC) developed with the special contribution of the European Heart Rhythm Association (EHRA) of the ESC. Eur Heart J 42(5):373–498
4. Gintant G, Sager PT, Stockbridge N (2016) Evolution of strategies to improve preclinical cardiac safety testing. Nat Rev Drug Discovery 15(7):457–471
5. Trayanova NA, Prakosa A (2024) Up digital and personal: how heart digital twins can transform heart patient care. Heart Rhythm 21(1):89–99
6. Oberman R, Shumway KR, Bhardwaj A (2023) Physiology cardiac. [Updated 2023 Jul 30]. In: StatPearls [Internet]. Treasure Island (FL): *StatPearls* Publishing; 2024 Jan. Available from https://www.ncbi.nlm.nih.gov/books/NBK526089/
7. Tse G (2016) Mechanisms of cardiac arrhythmias. J Arrhythmia 32(2):75–81
8. Heaton J, Goyal A (2023) Atrioventricular node. StatPearls Publishing, In StatPearls
9. Fogoros RN, Mandrola JM (2017) Fogoros' electrophysiologic testing. John Wiley & Sons
10. Antzelevitch C, Burashnikov A (2011) Overview of basic mechanisms of cardiac arrhythmia. Card Electrophysiol Clin 3(1):23–45
11. Frangogiannis NG (2021) Cardiac fibrosis. Cardiovasc Res 117(6):1450–1488
12. Moss AJ, Zareba W, Hall WJ, Klein H, Wilber DJ, Cannom DS, Andrews ML (2002) Prophylactic implantation of a defibrillator in patients with myocardial infarction and reduced ejection fraction. N Engl J Med 346(12):877–883
13. Schotten U, Verheule S, Kirchhof P, Goette A (2011) Pathophysiological mechanisms of atrial fibrillation: a translational appraisal. Physiol Rev 91(1):265–325
14. Yousuf O, Chrispin J, Tomaselli GF, Berger RD (2015) Clinical management and prevention of sudden cardiac death. Circ Res 116(12):2020–2040
15. Antiarrhythmics versus implantable defibrillators (AVID) Investigators (1997) A comparison of antiarrhythmic-drug therapy with implantable defibrillators in patients resuscitated from near-fatal ventricular arrhythmias. N Engl J Med 337(22):1576–1584
16. Prakosa A, Arevalo HJ, Deng D, Boyle PM, Nikolov PP, Ashikaga H, Trayanova NA (2018) Personalized virtual-heart technology for guiding the ablation of infarct-related ventricular tachycardia. Nat Biomed Eng 2(10):732–740
17. Josephson ME, Waxman HL, Cain ME, Gardner MJ, Buxton AE (1982) Ventricular activation during ventricular endocardial pacing. II. Role of pace-mapping to localize origin of ventricular tachycardia. Am J Cardiol 50(1):11–22
18. Rothman SA, Hsia HH, Cossu SF, Chmielewski IL, Buxton AE, Miller JM (1997) Radiofrequency catheter ablation of postinfarction ventricular tachycardia: long-term success and the significance of inducible nonclinical arrhythmias. Circulation 96(10):3499–3508
19. Corral-Acero J, Margara F, Marciniak M, Rodero C, Loncaric F, Feng Y, Lamata P (2020) The 'Digital Twin' to enable the vision of precision cardiology. Eur Heart J 41(48):4556–4564
20. Hodgkin AL, Huxley AF (1952) A quantitative description of membrane current and its application to conduction and excitation in nerve. J Physiol 117(4):500
21. Beeler GW, Reuter H (1977) Reconstruction of the action potential of ventricular myocardial fibres. J Physiol 268(1):177–210
22. Courtemanche M, Ramirez RJ, Nattel S (1998) Ionic mechanisms underlying human atrial action potential properties: insights from a mathematical model. Am J Physiol-Hear Circ Physiol 275(1):H301–H321
23. Biswas BN, Chatterjee S, Mukherjee SP, Pal S (2013) A discussion on Euler method: a review. Electron J Math Anal Appl 1(2):2090–2792
24. Neic A, Campos FO, Prassl AJ, Niederer SA, Bishop MJ, Vigmond EJ, Plank G (2017) Efficient computation of electrograms and ECGs in human whole heart simulations using a reaction-eikonal model. J Comput Phys 346:191–211
25. Clayton RH, Bernus O, Cherry EM, Dierckx H, Fenton FH, Mirabella L, Zhang H (2011) Models of cardiac tissue electrophysiology: progress, challenges and open questions. Prog Biophys Mol Biol 104(1–3):22–48
26. Keener J, Sneyd J (Eds.) (2009) Mathematical physiology: II: systems physiology. New York, NY, Springer New York
27. Bifulco SF, Akoum N, Boyle PM (2021) Translational applications of computational modelling for patients with cardiac arrhythmias. Heart 107(6):456–461
28. Zhang Y, Barocas VH, Berceli SA, Clancy CE, Eckmann DM, Garbey M, Trayanova NA (2016) Multi-scale modeling of the cardiovascular system: disease development, progression, and clinical intervention. Ann Biomed Eng 44:2642–2660
29. Dey D, Slomka PJ, Leeson P, Comaniciu D, Shrestha S, Sengupta PP, Marwick TH (2019) Artificial intelligence in cardiovascular imaging: JACC state-of-the-art review. J Am Coll Cardiol 73(11):1317–1335
30. Arevalo HJ, Vadakkumpadan F, Guallar E, Jebb A, Malamas P, Wu KC, Trayanova NA (2016) Arrhythmia risk stratification of patients after myocardial infarction using personalized heart models. Nat Commun 7(1):11437
31. Sung E, Prakosa A, Aronis KN et al (2020) Personalized digital-heart technology for ventricular tachycardia ablation targeting in hearts with infiltrating adiposity. Circ: Arrhythmia Electrophysiol 13(12):e008912

32. Boyle PM, Zghaib T, Zahid S, Ali RL, Deng D, Franceschi WH, Trayanova NA (2019) Computationally guided personalized targeted ablation of persistent atrial fibrillation. Nat Biomed Eng 3(11):870–879
33. Albatat M, Arevalo H, Bergsland J, Strøm V, Balasingham I, Odland HH (2021) Optimal pacing sites in cardiac resynchronization by left ventricular activation front analysis. Comput Biol Med 128:104159
34. Koopsen T, Gerrits W, van Osta N, van Loon T, Wouters P, Prinzen FW, Lumens J et al. (2024) Virtual pacing of a patient's digital twin to predict left ventricular reverse remodelling after cardiac resynchronization therapy. Eur 26(1):euae009
35. Bai W, Sinclair M, Tarroni G, Oktay O, Rajchl M, Vaillant G, Rueckert D (2018) Automated cardiovascular magnetic resonance image analysis with fully convolutional networks. J Cardiovasc Magn Reson 20(1):1–12
36. Ronneberger O, Fischer P, Brox T (2015) U-net: convolutional networks for biomedical image segmentation. In: Medical image computing and computer-assisted intervention–MICCAI 2015: 18th International conference, Munich, Germany, October 5–9, 2015, Proceedings, Part III 18 (pp 234–241). Springer International Publishing
37. Zhu Z, Xia Y, Shen W, Fishman E, Yuille A (2018) A 3D coarse-to-fine framework for volumetric medical image segmentation. In: 2018 international conference on 3D vision (3DV). IEEE, pp 682–690
38. Makela T, Clarysse P, Sipila O, Pauna N, Pham QC, Katila T, Magnin IE (2002) A review of cardiac image registration methods. IEEE Trans Med Imaging 21(9):1011–1021
39. Vigmond EJ, Dos Santos RW, Prassl AJ, Deo M, Plank G (2008) Solvers for the cardiac bidomain equations. Prog Biophys Mol Biol 96(1–3):3–18
40. Gillette K, Gsell MA, Strocchi M, Grandits T, Neic A, Manninger M, Plank G (2022) A personalized real-time virtual model of whole heart electrophysiology. Front Physiol 13:907190
41. Zhang YJ (2018) Geometric modeling and mesh generation from scanned images. Chapman and Hall/CRC
42. Bayer J, Prassl AJ, Pashaei A, Gomez JF, Frontera A, Neic A, Vigmond EJ (2018) Universal ventricular coordinates: a generic framework for describing position within the heart and transferring data. Med Image Anal 45:83–93
43. Roney CH, Pashaei A, Meo M, Dubois R, Boyle PM, Trayanova NA, Vigmond EJ (2019) Universal atrial coordinates applied to visualisation, registration and construction of patient specific meshes. Med Image Anal 55:65–75
44. Cárdenes R, Sebastian R, Soto-Iglesias D, Berruezo A, Camara O (2015) Estimation of Purkinje trees from electro-anatomical mapping of the left ventricle using minimal cost geodesics. Med Image Anal 24(1):52–62
45. Gillette K, Gsell MA, Prassl AJ, Karabelas E, Reiter U, Reiter G, Plank G (2021) A framework for the generation of digital twins of cardiac electrophysiology from clinical 12-leads ECGs. Med Image Anal 71:102080
46. Niederer SA, Kerfoot E, Benson AP, Bernabeu MO, Bernus O, Bradley C, Smith NP (2011) Verification of cardiac tissue electrophysiology simulators using an N-version benchmark. Philos Trans R Soc A: Math, Phys Eng Sci 369(1954):4331–4351
47. Plank G, Loewe A, Neic A, Augustin C, Huang YL, Gsell MA, Vigmond EJ (2021) The openCARP simulation environment for cardiac electrophysiology. Comput Methods Programs Biomed 208:106223
48. Stolarski T, Nakasone Y, Yoshimoto S (2018) Engineering analysis with ANSYS software. Butterworth-Heinemann
49. Shahriari B, Swersky K, Wang Z, Adams RP, De Freitas N (2015) Taking the human out of the loop: a review of Bayesian optimization. Proc IEEE 104(1):148–175
50. Nelder JA, Mead R (1965) A simplex method for function minimization. Comput J 7(4):308–313
51. Broyden CG (1970) The convergence of a class of double-rank minimization algorithms 1. General considerations. *IMA J Appl Math* 6(1):76–90
52. Bhagirath P, Campos FO, Postema PG, Kemme MJ, Wilde AA, Prassl AJ, Bishop MJ (2023) Arrhythmogenic vulnerability of re-entrant pathways in post-infarct ventricular tachycardia assessed by advanced computational modelling. Europace 25(9):euad198
53. Hwang M, Kwon SS, Wi J, Park M, Lee HS, Park JS, Pak HN (2014) Virtual ablation for atrial fibrillation in personalized in-silico three-dimensional left atrial modeling: comparison with clinical catheter ablation. Prog Biophys Mol Biol 116(1):40–47
54. Trayanova NA, Lyon A, Shade J, Heijman J (2024) Computational modeling of cardiac electrophysiology and arrhythmogenesis: toward clinical translation. Physiol Rev 104(3):1265–1333
55. Shim J, Hwang M, Song JS et al (2017) Virtual in-silico modeling guided catheter ablation predicts effective linear ablation lesion set for longstanding persistent atrial fibrillation: multicenter prospective randomized study. Front Physiol 8:792
56. Baek YS, Kwon OS, Lim B, Yang SY, Park JW, Yu HT et al. CUVIA-AF 2 investigators (2021) Clinical outcomes of computational virtual mapping-guided catheter ablation in patients with persistent atrial fibrillation: a multicenter prospective randomized clinical trial. Front Cardiovasc Med 8:772665
57. Clerx M, Collins P, De Lange E, Volders PG (2016) Myokit: a simple interface to cardiac cellular electrophysiology. Prog Biophys Mol Biol 120(1–3):100–114
58. Gray RA, Pathmanathan P (2018) Patient-specific cardiovascular computational modeling: diversity of personalization and challenges. J Cardiovasc Transl Res 11:80–88
59. Wu H, Ji P, Ma H, Xing L (2023) A comprehensive review of digital twin from the perspective of total process: data, models, networks and applications. Sensors 23(19):8306
60. Heijman J, Sutanto H, Crijns HJ, Nattel S, Trayanova NA (2021) Computational models of atrial fibrillation: achievements, challenges, and perspectives for improving clinical care. Cardiovasc Res 117(7):1682–1699

# Plasmonic Photothermal Therapy for Rapid and Total Eradication of Topical Gram-Negative Bacteria Infections

10

Satyajit Lenka, Deepak Kumar, Prachi Srivastava, Vivek Verma, Nagma Parveen, Tarun Gupta, and Manabendra Chandra

**Abstract**

Gram-negative bacterial infections pose a significant health challenge globally, particularly in wound care, where pathogens such as *Escherichia coli*, *Pseudomonas aeruginosa*, and *Acinetobacter baumannii* are prevalent. These infections are notorious for their resistance to conventional antibiotics and their ability to evade the immune response, leading to severe complications, including sepsis and high mortality rates. In India, these infections account for approximately 30% of hospital-acquired infections, highlighting the urgent need for innovative therapeutic strategies. This study investigates the efficacy of plasmonic photothermal therapy (PPTT) utilizing plasmonic nanoparticles (PNPs) to selectively target and eradicate Gram-negative bacteria. We demonstrate that PNPs, when exposed to near-infrared (NIR) laser irradiation, induce localized hyperthermia sufficient to destroy bacterial cells while sparing surrounding healthy tissue. Our results indicate that PNPs effectively bind to bacterial surfaces, promoting clustering and subsequent thermal destruction upon laser activation. In vitro assays reveal over 80% bacterial eradication within minutes of treatment without harming human red blood cells. This novel approach not only offers a viable alternative to traditional antibiotic therapies but also shows promise for enhancing wound healing outcomes, paving the way for future clinical trials and in vivo applications aimed at improving patient outcomes and reducing healthcare burdens associated with antibiotic resistance.

**Keywords**

Gram-negative bacteria · *E. coli* · Plasmonic photothermal therapy · Gold nanoparticles

## 10.1 Introduction

Gram-negative bacterial infections, particularly those affecting wound sites, represent a significant health burden in India and other parts of the world [1–3]. These infections, caused by pathogens such as *Escherichia coli*, *Pseudomonas aeruginosa*, and *Acinetobacter baumannii*, are known for their ability to evade the immune system and resist traditional antibiotic treatments, often leading to severe complications like bloodstream infections, sepsis, and, in many cases, death [4]. The prevalence of Gram-negative bacterial infections in healthcare settings is alarming, particularly in surgical site infections, diabetic foot ulcers, and burn wounds [5, 6]. In India, wound infections account for nearly 30% of all hospital-acquired infections, with Gram-negative bacteria being the most common. Data from healthcare reports indicate that among the Indian population, Gram-negative bacterial infections are a leading cause of mortality and morbidity. Surgical site infections affect about 30% of patients, with burn wounds and diabetic foot ulcers contributing to high mortality rates. Specifically, diabetic foot ulcers impact

S. Lenka · D. Kumar · P. Srivastava · V. Verma · N. Parveen · M. Chandra (✉)
Department of Chemistry, IIT Kanpur, Kanpur, India
e-mail: mchandra@iitk.ac.in

T. Gupta
Department of Civil Engineering, IIT Kanpur, Kanpur, India



S. Verma (ed.), *Technology and Innovation in Medical Sciences*, IITK Directions 7,
https://doi.org/10.1007/978-981-96-8606-3_10

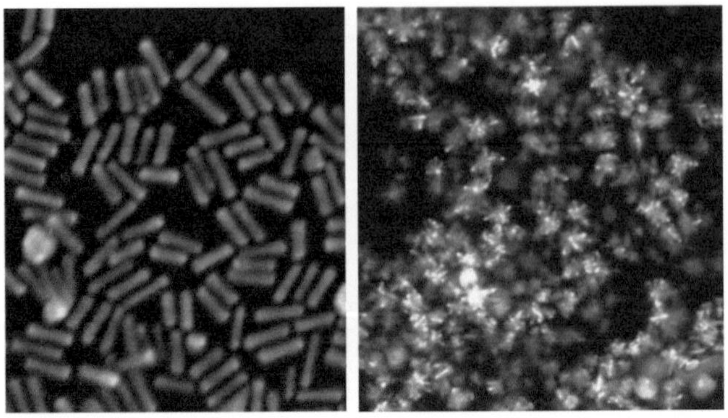

**Fig. 10.1** Electron microghaphs of prepared GNPs. Gold nanorod (left) and gold nanostar (right)

23% of the population, while burn wound infections contribute to 5.86% of cases [7]. These types of infections are not only difficult to treat but also frequently result in complications, leading to amputation in diabetic patients and prolonged hospital stays in burn patients. Mortality rates associated with these infections are disturbingly high, with some studies reporting death in 2.93% of the affected population. This underscores the need for an innovative and effective therapeutic strategy to combat these pathogens and reduce infection-related mortality. The challenge posed by these infections is further exacerbated by the emergence of multidrug-resistant (MDR) strains of Gram-negative bacteria [8]. As the World Health Organization (WHO) notes, 10 out of 12 high-priority pathogens requiring urgent development of new antibiotics are Gram-negative bacteria [9]. The mortality risk associated with these infections is highest in healthcare settings, where nearly 25% of patients are at risk of contracting MDR infections, with a mortality risk ranging from 50 to 80% in cases of sepsis and bloodstream infections [3, 10]. These statistics highlight the urgent need for alternative treatments that can overcome the limitations of current antibiotic therapies.

Plasmonic photothermal therapy (PPTT) is a promising and innovative solution to address this growing problem [11]. This novel treatment harnesses the power of plasmonic nanoparticles (PNPs; for example, gold nanoparticle or GNP), which can be engineered to selectively target and destroy Gram-negative bacteria [12–18]. The potential impact of PPTT is further emphasized by market opportunities in wound care, which are projected to grow significantly in the coming years. With the rise of antibiotic resistance and the high mortality risk associated with Gram-negative infections, there is a critical need for new therapies like PPTT [11, 13, 17–22]. This innovative approach could drastically reduce treatment times, improve patient outcomes, and alleviate the strain on healthcare systems by reducing the need for prolonged hospital stays and expensive treatments. Given the scale of the problem and the promising results of plasmonic photothermal therapy, this technique holds great potential for transforming the treatment of Gram-negative bacterial infections in wound care.

In this study, PPTT offers a two-step approach to effectively treat these infections. In the first step, gold nanoparticles are added to high density bacterial cells, either dispersed in water or attached to glass surface. Nanoparticles selectively bind to Gram-negative bacteria, and lead to the clustering of bacterial cells, while leaving host cells unaffected. This selective attachment prevents the bacteria from spreading and inhibits biofilm formation, a key defense mechanism of bacteria that makes them resistant to treatment. In the second step of the treatment, the continued application of NIR laser irradiation activates the gold nanoparticles. The particles absorb NIR light, causing a localized increase in temperature. This thermal effect is powerful enough to destroy the bacterial cells within minutes of laser exposure, while the surrounding host cells remain unharmed. This method ensures rapid bacterial eradication without the risk of damaging healthy tissue, which is a common side effect of traditional treatments like antibiotics or surgical debridement.

## 10.2 Result and Discussion

**PNP Synthesis and Characterization**: Gold nanorods and gold nanostars were synthesized using seed-mediated methods [23]. The structure and morphology were characterized using transmission electron microscopy (TEM) and scanning electron microscopy (SEM) (Fig. 10.1). The average dimensions of synthesized Gold nanorods and gold nanostars are provided in Table 10.1. We also synthesized gold nanospheres using sodium citrate reduction methods.

Next, we obtain the UV–visible absorption spectrum of Au nanoparticles. The LSPR maxima for nanorod and nanostars are observed at ~800 nm (Fig. 10.2). On the other hand, Au nanospheres show their typical absorption peak at around 520 nm. The strong absorption peak of the nanorod and the nanostars in the near-infrared (NIR) region indicates that they could convert

**Table 10.1** Size, ligand charge and LSPR maxima of the prepared PNPs

| GNP Shape | Size (nm) | Ligand charge | LSPR max (nm) |
|---|---|---|---|
| Nanosphere (NSP) | 82.15 ± 34.54 | Positive | ~520 |
| Nanorod (GNRs) | 87.31 ± 16.85 | Positive | ~800 |
| Nanostar (NSts) | 96.83 ± 29.26 | Positive | ~800 |

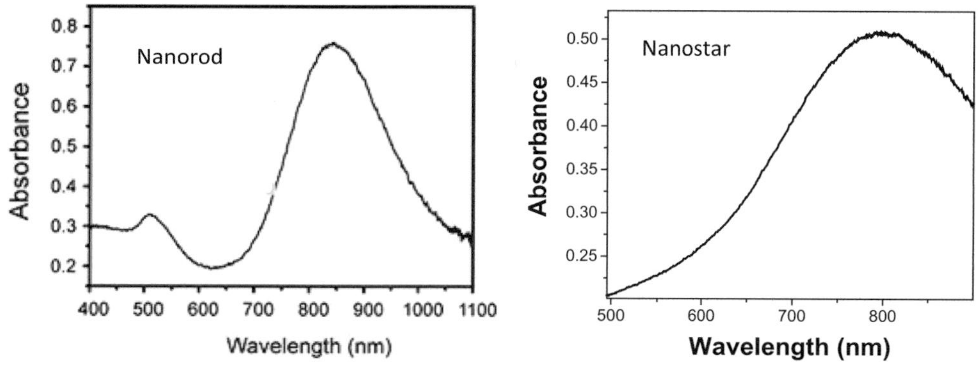


**Fig. 10.2** Vis-NIR spectra of gold nanorod and nanostar in aqueous solution

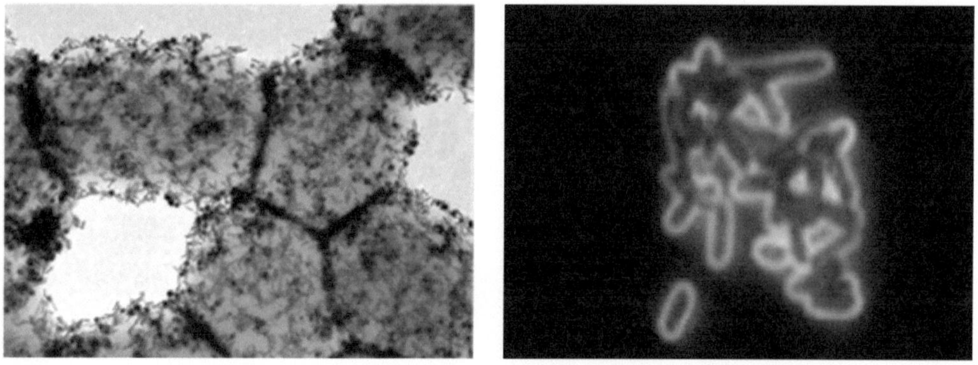

**Fig. 10.3** TEM and dark-field images showing surface attachment of GNPs and clustering of *E. coli* cells

the NIR light into heat via the decay of the localized surface plasmon resonance (LSPR) excitation [24, 25]. These two NIR absorbing anisotropic GNPs have the potential to be used for photothermal therapy. The 520 nm peak of Au nanospheres do not enable them to absorb light in the NIR region and thereby can act as a good control. Several capping agents (negatively charged, positively charged as well as neutral) were used to modify the surface. In this study, the capping agent was applied to enhance the stability of GNPs and most importantly, to aid in their attachment to Gram negative bacterial cells.

The photothermal properties of the synthesized nanoparticles were determined in aqueous solution. As expected aqueous solutions of nanorods and nanostars displayed the highest temperature elevation, making them the most effective candidate for plasmonic photothermal therapy.

**Selective attachment of the PNPs to Gram-negative bacteria cells**: In the next step, *E. coli* (MC4100) cells were subjected to GNP exposure. GNPs functionalized with positively charged ligands show tendency to get attached onto the bacterial surface and lead to clustering of the *E. coli* cells (Fig. 10.3). The UV–visible spectroscopy shows a complementary result with the microscopy results. The absorbance spectra show a red shift in the case of the GNRs attached to *E.coli* bacteria and form the clusters w.r.t the only GNRs in the PBS buffer.

The UV-visible spectra of the different concentrations of GNRs with the E. coli LPS show a peak at around 800 nm, the same peak we observed in the case of only GNRs solution in PBS, but the absorbance is low which confirmed that the free GNRs low in the number, i.e., they have bound on the surface of the E. coli LPS. However, this was not the case in the presence of any concentration of E. coli phospholipids. Further, this observation was confirmed by the TEM image of the E. coli bacterial cells attached to the GNRs (Fig. 10.3), where we can see that the bacteria cell was completely covered and clustered with the GNRs.

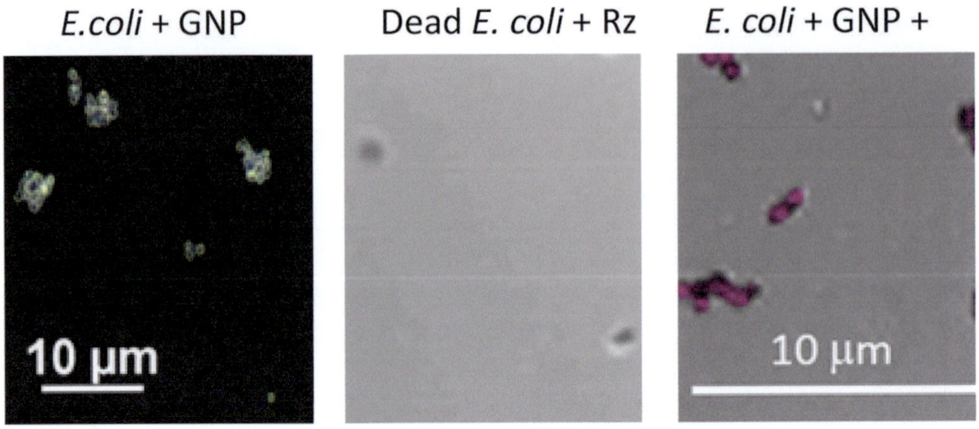


**Fig. 10.4** Resazurin assay. Combined confocal and DIC images of dead *E. coli* cells (left) and GNP treated *E. coli* clusters before any laser irradiation. Dead E. coli cells act as control

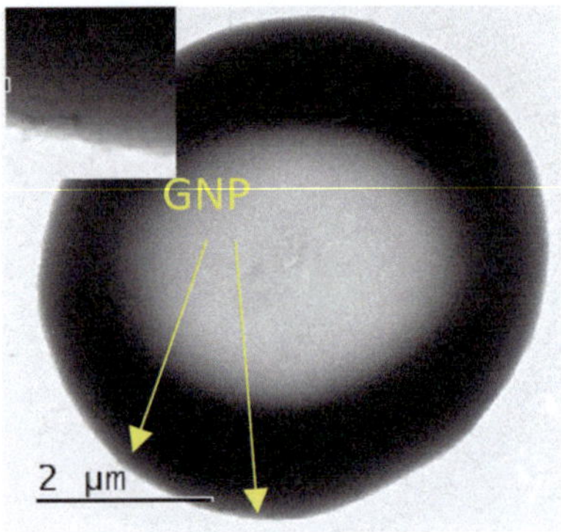


**Fig. 10.5** TEM image of hRBC treated with GNPs. Negligible binding/uptake of GNPs by hRBC is obvious

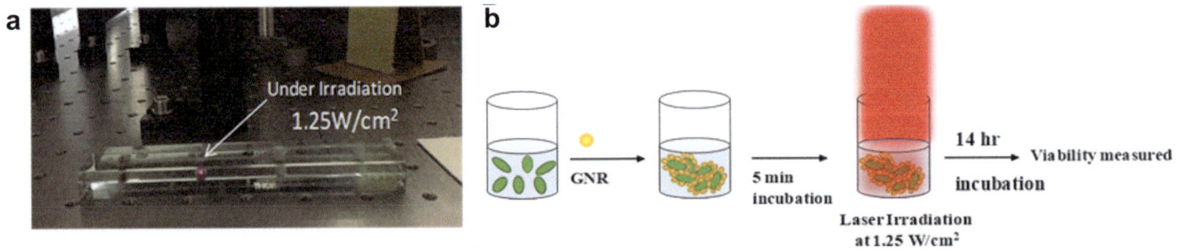


**Fig. 10.6** **(a)** Built-in-house multi-well glass block for plasmonic photothermal study in solution phase. **(b)** Scheme of plasmonic photothermal study in solution phase

We checked the effect of GNP treatment on the viability of the *E. coli* cells. The resazurin assays (Fig. 10.4) reveal that the GNP attached *E. coli* cells are metabolically active. This suggest that GNP treatment is nonlethal to *E. coli* cells. At this point, we subjected human red blood cells (hRBC) to the GNP treatment to check whether GNPs attach onto host cells and damage them. This is important since at the infection site the GNPs will always have contact with blood cells, any toxic effect on the blood cells should be always taken care of. We found that GNP attachment to hRBCs is negligible (Fig. 10.5). Also, no discernible hemolysis was detected. This indicates that in presence of host cells, GNP selectively binds to Gram-negative bacteria cell.

**Photothermal therapy by NIR Laser at solution phase**: Next, only *E. coli* cells as well as cells treated with GNPs were irradiated with 800 nm laser for the same time. A specially designed multi-well glass block was used for this purpose (Fig. 10.6a). The bacteria and the 2 nM concentration of GNPs were suspended in the aqueous solution and incubated for 5 min. Next, the samples were irradiated with 800 nm laser for up to 10 min and then they were kept for 14 h. After 14 h, the bacterial cell viability was measured (Scheme Fig. 10.6b).

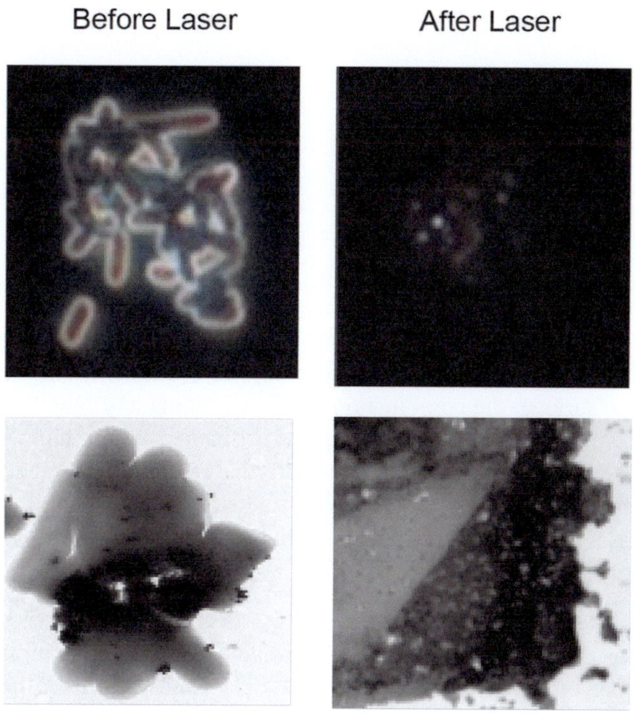


**Fig. 10.7** Optical dark-field images (top panel) and TEM images (bottom panel) of GNP treated E. coli cells before and after irradiation in aqueous dispersion

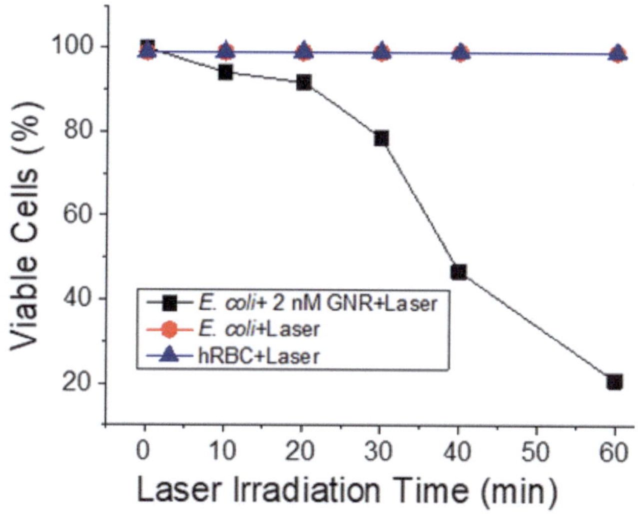


**Fig. 10.8** Viable cells as a function of laser irradiation time

Gold nanorods and nanostars displayed excellent bacterial killing efficiency upon laser irradiation as clearly evident from the optical dark-field as well as TEM images (Fig. 10.7). Interestingly, more than 80% of the *E. coli* cells ($10^9$ cells/ml) were destroyed within 50 min of laser exposure.

The anisotropic GNPs show the most significant reduction in *E. coli* viability, with only 20% viable bacterial cells remaining upon prolong irradiation (Figs. 10.7 and 10.8). This fast bacterial death is because of the rapid temperature rise in the proximity of GNPs following LSPR photoexcitation. Note that at the same concentration, the spherical nanoparticles showed extremely low photothermal damage to *E. coli* cells.

**Photothermal therapy by NIR Laser on the surface**: To mimic the tropical wound infection, we carried out the GNP induced photothermal experiments (similar to what have been discussed in the previous section) but on the *E. coli* cells attached to glass surface [8, 26].

(Scheme in Fig. 10.9) shows the pictorial representation of our experiment at the surface level. Here we show that the GNPs are particularly effective in killing high density *E. coli* cells fixed onto a surface. The fluorescence micrograph of fixed

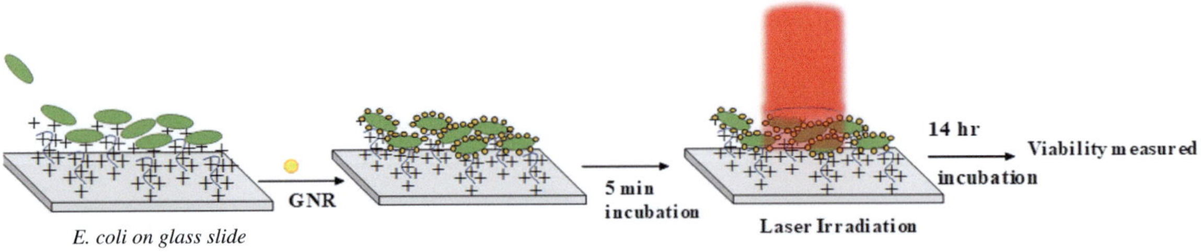


**Fig. 10.9** Scheme of plasmonic photothermal study on *E. coli* immobilized on glass surface

*E. coli* treated with GNR before the laser treatment. The decimation of the *E. coli* cells after laser irradiation is obvious. At the surface, the combination of GNR binding and NIR laser irradiation damaged 80% of bacteria within 5 min, instead of 50 min in solution. As a control experiment, we used human RBC treated with GNR before and after NIR laser irradiation to check this effect on the normal cells and we observed that before and after laser treatment on this combination doesn't change the cell viability. The dark field microscopy shows that in the absence of the GNR, the *E. coli* cells irradiated with the NIR laser do not show clustering and damage, however in the presence of GNR we can see the clusters were destroyed completely after irradiating the laser.

**Conclusion and Future Prospects**: This preliminary study confirms the potential of plasmonic therapy as an effective strategy for the eradication of Gram-negative bacteria and the enhancement of wound healing. Plasmonic nanorods and nanostars showed superior photothermal efficiency and bacterial killing capability without affecting the normal cells. Additionally, the rapid destruction of high density bacteria cells attached on glass surface providing a promising treatment modality for infected wounds and faster wound healing. Future work will focus on the further optimization and followed by test on animal wounds and the clinical trials.

**Acknowledgements** We would like to sincerely thank Dr. Anindita Gayen for her valuable discussions, insightful suggestions, and constructive feedback, which significantly contributed to the development of this work. This work is supported by the Gangwal School of Medical Sciences and Technology, IIT Kanpur, Kanpur.

**Author Contribution** MC conceived the study and designed the experiments; SL, DK, PS and VV carried out the experiments, performed the data analysis and interpretation. The manuscript was written with the contributions of all authors. All authors have approved the final version of the manuscript.

**Notes** The authors have no competing financial and commercial interests.

## References

1. Breijyeh Z, Jubeh B, Karaman R (2020) Resistance of gram-negative bacteria to current antibacterial agents and approaches to resolve it. Molecules. MDPI AG March 2 2020. https://doi.org/10.3390/molecules25061340
2. Murray CJ, Ikuta KS, Sharara F, Swetschinski L, Robles Aguilar G, Gray A et al (2022) Global burden of bacterial antimicrobial resistance in 2019: a systematic analysis. The Lancet 399(10325):629–655. https://doi.org/10.1016/S0140-6736(21)02724-0
3. Ikuta KS, Swetschinski LR, Aguilar GR, Sharara F, Mestrovic T, Gray AP et al (2022) Global mortality associated with 33 bacterial pathogens in 2019: a systematic analysis for the Global Burden of Disease Study 2019. Lancet 400(10369):2221–2248. https://doi.org/10.1016/S0140-6736(22)02185-7
4. Mancuso G, Midiri A, Gerace E, Biondo C (2021) Bacterial antibiotic resistance: the most critical pathogens. Pathogens. MDPI October 1 2021. https://doi.org/10.3390/pathogens10101310
5. Goh TC, Goh TC, Bajuri MY, Nadarajah SC, Abdul Rashid AH, Baharuddin S, et al (2020) Clinical and bacteriological profile of diabetic foot infections in tertiary care. J Foot Ankle Res 13(1). https://doi.org/10.1186/s13047-020-00406-y
6. Baig MS, Banu A, Zehravi M, Rana R, Burle SS, Khan SL, et al (2022) An overview of diabetic foot ulcers and associated problems with special emphasis on treatments with antimicrobials. Life. MDPI July 1 2022. https://doi.org/10.3390/life12071054
7. Sethuram L, Thomas J, Mukherjee A, Chandrasekaran N (2022) A review on contemporary nanomaterial-based therapeutics for the treatment of diabetic foot ulcers (DFUs) with special reference to the Indian scenario. Nanoscale Advances R Soc Chem. https://doi.org/10.1039/d1na00859e
8. Qin S, Xiao W, Zhou C, Pu Q, Deng X, Lan L, et al (2022) Pseudomonas aeruginosa: pathogenesis, virulence factors, antibiotic resistance, interaction with host, technology advances and emerging therapeutics. Signal Transduct Target Ther, Springer Nature Dec 1 2022. https://doi.org/10.1038/s41392-022-01056-1

9. Asokan GV, Ramadhan T, Ahmed E, Sanad H (2019) WHO global priority pathogens list: a bibliometric analysis of medline-pubmed for knowledge mobilization to infection prevention and control practices in Bahrain. Oman Med J. Oman Medical Specialty Board May 1 2019, pp 184–193. https://doi.org/10.5001/omj.2019.37
10. Gandra S, Tseng KK, Arora A, Bhowmik B, Robinson ML, Panigrahi B et al (2019) The mortality burden of multidrug-resistant pathogens in India: a retrospective. Obs Study Clin Infect Dis 69(4):563–570. https://doi.org/10.1093/cid/ciy955
11. Zharov VP, Galitovsky V, Viegas M (2003) Photothermal detection of local thermal effects during selective nanophotothermolysis. Appl Phys Lett 83(24):4897–4899. https://doi.org/10.1063/1.1632546
12. Pajerski W, Ochonska D, Brzychczy-Wloch M, Indyka P, Jarosz M, Golda-Cepa M, et al (2019) Attachment efficiency of gold nanoparticles by Gram-positive and Gram-negative bacterial strains governed by surface charges. J Nanoparticle Res 21(8). https://doi.org/10.1007/s11051-019-4617-z
13. Huang X, Jain PK, El-Sayed IH, El-Sayed MA (2008) Plasmonic photothermal therapy (PPTT) using gold nanoparticles. Lasers Med Sci, pp 217–228. https://doi.org/10.1007/s10103-007-0470-x
14. Pissuwan D, Valenzuela SM, Cortie MB (n.d.) Therapeutic possibilities of plasmonically heated gold nanoparticles. www.tcrt.com
15. Hegde M, Pai P, Shetty MG, Babitha KS (2022) Gold nanoparticle based biosensors for rapid pathogen detection: a review. Environ Nanotechnol, Monit Manag, Elsevier B.V. Dec 1 2022. https://doi.org/10.1016/j.enmm.2022.100756
16. Tian EK, Wang Y, Ren R, Zheng W, Liao W (2021) Gold nanoparticle: recent progress on its antibacterial applications and mechanisms. J Nanomater. Hindawi Limited. https://doi.org/10.1155/2021/2501345
17. Gharatape A, Davaran S, Salehi R, Hamishehkar H (2016) Engineered gold nanoparticles for photothermal cancer therapy and bacteria killing. RSC Adv 6(112):111482–111516. https://doi.org/10.1039/c6ra18760a
18. Zharov VP, Mercer KE, Galitovskaya EN, Smeltzer MS (2006) Photothermal nanotherapeutics and nanodiagnostics for selective killing of bacteria targeted with gold nanoparticles. Biophys J 90(2):619–627. https://doi.org/10.1529/biophysj.105.061895
19. Chiang WL, Lin TT, Sureshbabu R, Chia WT, Hsiao HC, Liu HY et al (2015) A rapid drug release system with a NIR light-activated molecular switch for dual-modality photothermal/antibiotic treatments of subcutaneous abscesses. J Control Release 199:53–62. https://doi.org/10.1016/j.jconrel.2014.12.011
20. Von Maltzahn G, Park JH, Agrawal A, Bandaru NK, Das SK, Sailor MJ et al (2009) Computationally guided photothermal tumor therapy using long-circulating gold nanorod antennas. Can Res 69(9):3892–3900. https://doi.org/10.1158/0008-5472.CAN-08-4242
21. Yu Q, Li J, Zhang Y, Wang Y, Liu L, Li M (2016) Inhibition of gold nanoparticles (AuNPs) on pathogenic biofilm formation and invasion to host cells. Sci Rep 6:26667. https://doi.org/10.1038/srep26667
22. Kim SE, Lee BR, Lee H, Jo SD, Kim H, Won YY et al (2017) Near-infrared plasmonic assemblies of gold nanoparticles with multimodal function for targeted cancer theragnosis. Sci Rep 7(1). https://doi.org/10.1038/s41598-017-17714-2
23. Wei MZ, Deng TS, Zhang Q, Cheng Z, Li S (2021) Seed-mediated synthesis of gold nanorods at low concentrations of CTAB. ACS Omega 6(13):9188–9195. https://doi.org/10.1021/acsomega.1c00510
24. Ha M, Kim JH, You M, Li Q, Fan C, Nam JM (2019) Multicomponent plasmonic nanoparticles: from heterostructured nanoparticles to colloidal composite nanostructures. Chem Rev. American Chemical Society Dec 26 2019, pp 12208–12278. https://doi.org/10.1021/acs.chemrev.9b00234
25. Zheng J, Cheng X, Zhang H, Bai X, Ai R, Shao L et al (2021) Gold nanorods: the most versatile plasmonic nanoparticles. Chem Rev. American Chemical Society Nov 10 2021, pp 13342–13453. https://doi.org/10.1021/acs.chemrev.1c00422
26. Haaber J, Cohn MT, Frees D, Andersen TJ, Ingmer H (2012) Planktonic aggregates of Staphylococcus aureus protect against common antibiotics. PLoS ONE 7(7). https://doi.org/10.1371/journal.pone.0041075

MIX
Papier aus verantwortungsvollen Quellen
Paper from responsible sources
FSC® C105338

If you have any concerns about our products,
you can contact us on
**ProductSafety@springernature.com**

In case Publisher is established outside the EU,
the EU authorized representative is:
**Springer Nature Customer Service Center GmbH**
**Europaplatz 3, 69115 Heidelberg, Germany**

Printed by Libri Plureos GmbH
in Hamburg, Germany